I0422538

TABLE OF CONTENTS

- Recognizing the symptoms and seeking medical help
- Diagnostic criteria and tests used for PCOS diagnosis
- Differential diagnoses and conditions to rule out
- Importance of early detection and intervention

Chapter 5: Managing PCOS: Medical Approaches

- Pharmacological treatments for symptom management
- Hormonal birth control options and their benefits
- Insulin-sensitizing medications and their role
- Managing infertility and assisted reproductive techniques

Chapter 6: Lifestyle Modifications and Self-Care

- The impact of diet and nutrition on PCOS
- Exercise and physical activity recommendations

- Stress management techniques and their significance
- Importance of sleep and maintaining a healthy routine

Chapter 7: Fertility and Pregnancy with PCOS
- Understanding ovulation and optimizing chances of conception
- PCOS-related challenges in pregnancy
- Managing gestational diabetes and other complications
- Postpartum considerations and long-term health planning

Chapter 8: Emotional Well-being and PCOS
- Addressing the emotional impact of PCOS
- Coping strategies for dealing with stress and anxiety
- Support systems: family, friends, and mental health professionals
- Building resilience and maintaining a positive outlook

Chapter 9: PCOS-Related Health Risks

- Long-term health risks: cardiovascular issues, diabetes, and more
- Regular health check-ups and monitoring
- Strategies for minimizing risks through lifestyle changes

Chapter 10: Research and Future Directions
- Current scientific research on PCOS
- Emerging treatments and interventions
- Advocacy and awareness initiatives
- The road ahead: hope for women with PCOS

Chapter 1: Introduction to PCOS

Definition and basics of Polycystic Ovary Syndrome (PCOS)

Polycystic Ovary Syndrome (PCOS) is a common hormonal disorder that affects people with ovaries, typically during their reproductive years. It is characterized by a combination of symptoms that can vary in severity and presentation. The term "polycystic" refers to the appearance of the ovaries, which may have multiple small cysts on their surface.

Key features of PCOS include:
1. Irregular Menstrual Cycles: Women with PCOS often experience irregular or infrequent menstrual cycles, which can make it difficult to predict ovulation and plan for pregnancy.

2. Elevated Androgens: Androgens are often referred to as "male hormones," although they are present in both sexes. People with PCOS may have higher levels of androgens, which can lead to symptoms like acne, excessive facial or body hair growth (hirsutism), and male-pattern baldness.

3. Ovulatory Dysfunction: Due to hormonal imbalances, some individuals with PCOS may not ovulate regularly or at all. This can result in difficulty getting pregnant.

4. Polycystic Ovaries: Ovaries of individuals with PCOS are often enlarged and contain multiple small follicles, which are sacs that contain immature eggs. Despite the name, these "cysts" are not the same as the fluid-filled cysts associated with other conditions.

5. Insulin Resistance: Many people with PCOS have insulin resistance, a condition where the body's cells do not respond effectively to insulin. This can lead to high levels of insulin in the blood, contributing to weight gain and metabolic issues.

6. Weight Gain: Weight gain and difficulty losing weight are common among individuals with PCOS, in part due to insulin resistance and hormonal imbalances.

It's important to note that the presentation of PCOS can vary widely, and not all individuals will experience all of these features. Diagnosis is typically made based on a combination of symptoms, medical history, physical examination, and sometimes additional tests such as blood tests and ultrasound imaging.

PCOS can have a significant impact on a person's physical and emotional well-being. Management approaches often involve a combination of lifestyle changes, medication, and sometimes assisted reproductive techniques for those struggling with fertility. Regular medical check-ups and ongoing communication with healthcare professionals are crucial for effectively managing PCOS and its associated health concerns.

Historical context and early recognition

The historical context of Polycystic Ovary Syndrome (PCOS) traces back several decades, with its recognition and understanding evolving over time. Here's a brief overview of the historical context and early recognition of PCOS:

Early Observations:

- The earliest documented cases that could potentially be attributed to PCOS date back

to the 18th and 19th centuries, but the condition was not well understood at that time.
- In the mid-20th century, medical professionals started observing a constellation of symptoms including irregular menstrual cycles, excessive hair growth, and enlarged ovaries during surgical procedures. However, these observations weren't always connected to a single syndrome.

The Stein-Leventhal Syndrome:
- In 1935, American gynecologists Irving F. Stein, Sr. and Michael L. Leventhal published a study that described seven women with amenorrhea (absence of menstrual periods), hirsutism (excessive hair growth), and enlarged ovaries with multiple cysts.
- They referred to this condition as "the syndrome of polycystic ovaries" and associated it with infertility.
- The syndrome was later known as the "Stein-Leventhal syndrome."

Evolution of Understanding:
- The 1980s marked a pivotal period when researchers began to recognize the hormonal and metabolic components of PCOS, linking it to insulin resistance and androgen excess.
- The National Institutes of Health (NIH) sponsored a conference in 1990 to establish diagnostic criteria for PCOS. This conference led to the Rotterdam criteria, which are still used today.

Contemporary Recognition and Awareness:
- PCOS gained increasing recognition in the 21st century as more research highlighted its prevalence and impact on women's health.
- Advances in medical imaging and technology made it easier to visualize the characteristic ovarian features of PCOS.
- Improved understanding of hormonal imbalances and insulin resistance led to more targeted treatment options.

In recent years, efforts have been made to raise awareness about PCOS and provide accurate information to both healthcare professionals and the general public. PCOS awareness months, research initiatives, and advocacy campaigns have contributed to a better understanding of the condition and its management.

Early recognition of PCOS is crucial for timely diagnosis and effective management. While historical observations laid the foundation, ongoing research and awareness efforts continue to shape our understanding of PCOS and improve the lives of those affected by it.

Prevalence and demographics

Polycystic Ovary Syndrome (PCOS) is one of the most common hormonal disorders affecting people with ovaries, and its prevalence varies among different populations and age groups. Here's an overview of the prevalence and demographics of PCOS:

Prevalence:
- PCOS is estimated to affect around 5% to 15% of women of reproductive age globally. However, the exact prevalence can vary depending on factors such as diagnostic criteria, study population, and geographic location.

Demographics:
- PCOS can affect individuals of all ethnicities and races. It's important to note that while it's commonly associated with women, PCOS can also affect transgender and non-binary individuals who have ovaries.
- The condition often becomes apparent during adolescence, with symptoms such as irregular periods and acne emerging in the teenage years. However, it can also be diagnosed later in life, especially when

individuals seek medical attention due to fertility concerns or other related symptoms.

- PCOS tends to run in families, suggesting a genetic component. If a close female family member has PCOS, there might be an increased risk of developing the condition.

Impact on Different Age Groups:
- Adolescents: PCOS can be particularly challenging for teenagers, as the hormonal and physical changes during puberty may exacerbate the symptoms. Early diagnosis and management are important to help alleviate distress and support healthy development.
- Reproductive Age: Many women with PCOS are diagnosed during their reproductive years, often when they face difficulties with menstrual irregularities, fertility issues, and other related symptoms.
- Perimenopause and Beyond: PCOS symptoms may change with age. Menstrual

irregularities might improve, but other aspects such as insulin resistance and cardiovascular risks might become more prominent.

Global Variations:
- PCOS prevalence can vary based on geographic regions and ethnic backgrounds. It has been reported to be more common in South Asian and Middle Eastern populations, but it is present in diverse populations across the world.

As understanding of PCOS continues to evolve, researchers are investigating its prevalence and impact in different populations. Early diagnosis and appropriate management are essential to address the various symptoms and potential long-term health risks associated with PCOS, ensuring better quality of life and health outcomes for those affected.

Common symptoms and diagnostic criteria

Common Symptoms of PCOS:

1. Irregular Menstrual Cycles: Women with PCOS often experience irregular or infrequent menstrual periods, which can range from missed periods to heavy and prolonged bleeding.

2. Androgen Excess: Elevated levels of androgens (male hormones) can lead to symptoms such as hirsutism (excessive hair growth on the face, chest, or back), acne, and male-pattern baldness.

3. Ovulatory Dysfunction: Irregular or absent ovulation can cause infertility or difficulties in conceiving. Some individuals may also experience unpredictable ovulation.

4. Polycystic Ovaries: Enlarged ovaries with multiple small cysts can be detected through medical imaging. However, the presence of these cysts is not always necessary for a PCOS diagnosis.

5. Insulin Resistance: Many people with PCOS have insulin resistance, which can lead to weight gain, difficulty losing weight, and an increased risk of type 2 diabetes.

6. Weight Gain: Weight gain and difficulty managing weight are common among individuals with PCOS, often due to hormonal imbalances and insulin resistance.

7. Skin Changes: In addition to acne, dark patches of skin, known as acanthosis nigricans, might appear in areas like the neck, armpits, or groin.

8. Mood Disturbances: Some individuals with PCOS might experience mood swings, anxiety, and depression, possibly related to hormonal fluctuations and the emotional impact of the condition.

Diagnostic Criteria:
Diagnosing PCOS involves assessing a combination of symptoms, medical history,

physical examination, and sometimes additional tests. There are different sets of diagnostic criteria, including those from the Rotterdam criteria and the Androgen Excess Society (AES) criteria. According to the Rotterdam criteria, a diagnosis of PCOS can be made if at least two of the following three criteria are met:

1. Oligo-ovulation or Anovulation: Irregular or absent menstrual cycles due to ovulatory dysfunction.
2. Clinical and/or Biochemical Signs of Hyperandrogenism: This could include hirsutism, acne, androgenic alopecia (male-pattern baldness), or elevated levels of androgens in blood tests.
3. Polycystic Ovaries: Presence of multiple small cysts on one or both ovaries, as visualized through ultrasound.

It's important to note that a comprehensive evaluation by a healthcare professional is necessary for an accurate diagnosis. Other conditions with similar symptoms, such as thyroid disorders and adrenal conditions, should be ruled out before arriving at a PCOS diagnosis.

Regular health check-ups, open communication with a healthcare provider, and a holistic approach to managing PCOS symptoms can significantly improve quality of life and mitigate potential long-term health risks associated with the condition.

Chapter 2: The Science Behind PCOS

Hormonal Imbalances and Insulin Resistance in PCOS

Hormonal Imbalances:
Polycystic Ovary Syndrome (PCOS) is characterized by disruptions in hormonal regulation. Some of the key hormonal imbalances include:

1. Androgens: Individuals with PCOS often have elevated levels of androgens, which are typically considered male hormones. This excess androgen production can lead to symptoms such as hirsutism (excessive hair growth), acne, and male-pattern baldness.

2. Estrogens: Disruptions in the balance between androgens and estrogens can lead to irregular menstrual cycles and anovulation (lack of ovulation).

3. Luteinizing Hormone (LH): Increased levels of LH relative to follicle-stimulating hormone (FSH) contribute to the

development of ovarian cysts, irregular ovulation, and increased androgen production.

4. Insulin: While insulin is not typically considered a sex hormone, its role in PCOS is significant. Insulin resistance is a common feature of PCOS and contributes to hormonal imbalances.

Insulin Resistance:
Insulin resistance occurs when the body's cells do not respond properly to insulin, a hormone that helps regulate blood sugar levels. In PCOS, insulin resistance has several implications:

1. Hyperinsulinemia: The body compensates for insulin resistance by producing more insulin. Elevated insulin levels can stimulate the ovaries to produce more androgens, worsening the hormonal imbalance.

2. Weight Gain: Insulin resistance can lead to weight gain or difficulty in losing weight. Fat cells are sensitive to insulin, and excess weight can exacerbate insulin resistance.

3. Impact on Ovulation: Insulin resistance can interfere with normal ovulation, contributing to irregular menstrual cycles and fertility issues.

4. Increased Risk of Type 2 Diabetes: Long-term insulin resistance can increase the risk of developing type 2 diabetes. This risk is higher in individuals with PCOS.

5. Metabolic Syndrome: Insulin resistance, along with other factors like high blood pressure and abnormal cholesterol levels, can contribute to the development of metabolic syndrome.

Managing Hormonal Imbalances and Insulin Resistance:

Addressing hormonal imbalances and insulin resistance is a critical aspect of managing PCOS:

- Lifestyle Changes: Adopting a healthy lifestyle that includes regular exercise and a balanced diet can improve insulin sensitivity, assist in weight management, and help regulate hormonal imbalances.

- Medications: Medications can be prescribed to help regulate menstrual cycles, reduce androgen levels, and improve insulin sensitivity. These may include hormonal contraceptives, anti-androgen medications, and insulin-sensitizing drugs.

- Weight Management: Achieving and maintaining a healthy weight can significantly improve insulin sensitivity and reduce the severity of PCOS symptoms.

- Dietary Choices: A low-glycemic-index diet that focuses on complex carbohydrates, lean proteins, and healthy fats can help manage blood sugar levels and insulin resistance.

- Regular Monitoring: Routine medical check-ups and blood tests are important for tracking insulin levels, blood sugar, and other metabolic indicators.

- Collaboration with Healthcare Providers: Working closely with healthcare professionals, such as endocrinologists, gynecologists, and dietitians, can ensure a comprehensive approach to managing PCOS.

Managing hormonal imbalances and insulin resistance can lead to improved symptom control, better overall health, and a reduced risk of long-term complications associated with PCOS.

Role of androgens and their impact

Androgens are a group of hormones that are commonly referred to as "male hormones," although they are present in both males and females. In Polycystic Ovary Syndrome (PCOS), elevated levels of androgens play a significant role in the development of various symptoms and complications. Here's an overview of the role of androgens and their impact in PCOS:

Role of Androgens:
- Androgens, including testosterone, dihydrotestosterone (DHT), and dehydroepiandrosterone (DHEA), are produced by the ovaries and adrenal glands in females.
- In PCOS, there is an overproduction of androgens, contributing to the hormonal imbalance observed in the condition.

Impact of Elevated Androgens in PCOS:
1. Hirsutism: Excessive hair growth in areas where males typically grow hair (face, chest, back) is a common symptom of elevated androgens in PCOS. This can have a

significant impact on self-esteem and body image.

2. Acne: Elevated androgens can lead to increased sebum production in the skin, causing acne and oily skin.

3. Male-Pattern Baldness: Androgens can contribute to hair thinning and hair loss similar to male-pattern baldness.

4. Menstrual Irregularities: High androgen levels can disrupt the balance between androgens and estrogens, leading to irregular menstrual cycles and anovulation (lack of ovulation).

5. Ovulatory Dysfunction: Androgen excess can contribute to the suppression of normal ovulatory processes, leading to fertility issues and difficulty conceiving.

6. Insulin Resistance: Androgens are believed to worsen insulin resistance, which is common in PCOS. This contributes to weight gain and metabolic disturbances.

7. Cardiovascular Risk: Elevated androgens have been associated with an increased risk of cardiovascular issues, including high blood pressure and abnormal cholesterol levels.

8. Psychological Impact: The physical symptoms caused by androgen excess can lead to psychological distress, affecting self-confidence and emotional well-being.

Managing Androgen Levels in PCOS: Managing the impact of elevated androgens is an important aspect of PCOS treatment:

- Hormonal Birth Control: Oral contraceptives that contain estrogen and a progestin can help regulate androgen levels, leading to improvements in hirsutism, acne, and menstrual irregularities.

- Anti-Androgen Medications: Medications that block the effects of androgens or reduce their production can be prescribed to manage hirsutism and other related symptoms.

- Lifestyle Changes: Lifestyle modifications such as weight management through exercise and a balanced diet can help improve androgen levels and insulin sensitivity.

- Insulin-Sensitizing Drugs: Medications that improve insulin sensitivity can indirectly help manage androgen levels by addressing insulin resistance.

- Topical Treatments: Topical creams or treatments can be used to manage hirsutism and acne, targeting specific affected areas.

- Medical Monitoring: Regular medical check-ups and blood tests are important for monitoring androgen levels and assessing the effectiveness of treatment.

Balancing androgen levels is essential not only for symptom management but also for reducing the risk of long-term health complications associated with PCOS. A personalized treatment plan, tailored to individual needs and symptoms, is crucial for effective management of elevated androgens in PCOS.

Ovulatory dysfunction and its consequences

Ovulatory dysfunction is a key feature of Polycystic Ovary Syndrome (PCOS), and it refers to the disruption or irregularity of the normal ovulation process. Ovulation is the release of a mature egg from the ovaries, which is essential for reproductive health. In PCOS, ovulatory dysfunction can have various consequences that impact fertility, menstrual cycles, and overall health. Here's an overview of ovulatory dysfunction and its consequences in PCOS:

Consequences of Ovulatory Dysfunction:

1. Infertility: Irregular or absent ovulation is a common cause of infertility in women with PCOS. Without regular

ovulation, the opportunity for fertilization and conception is limited.

2. Irregular Menstrual Cycles: Ovulatory dysfunction contributes to irregular menstrual cycles. Women with PCOS may experience longer or shorter cycles, heavy or unpredictable bleeding, or even months without a period.

3. Anovulation: Anovulation refers to the absence of ovulation. This can lead to a lack of menstruation altogether, making it challenging to predict fertility and conceive.

4. Difficulty Predicting Fertile Period: Women with PCOS may have difficulty predicting their fertile window due to irregular or absent ovulation. This can complicate family planning efforts.

5. Risk of Endometrial Hyperplasia: Prolonged periods without ovulation can lead to overgrowth of the uterine lining (endometrial hyperplasia), increasing the

risk of abnormal bleeding and potentially contributing to endometrial cancer.

6. Hormonal Imbalance: Ovulatory dysfunction contributes to hormonal imbalances, including elevated androgens and disrupted ratios of estrogen and progesterone. This can lead to various symptoms such as hirsutism, acne, and mood disturbances.

Managing Ovulatory Dysfunction in PCOS: Addressing ovulatory dysfunction is important for managing the associated consequences and improving overall reproductive and hormonal health:

- Lifestyle Changes: Lifestyle modifications such as maintaining a healthy weight through balanced nutrition and regular exercise can help improve ovulation and overall fertility.

- Hormonal Birth Control: Oral contraceptives containing estrogen and progestin can regulate menstrual cycles, improve hormonal balance, and manage symptoms associated with ovulatory dysfunction.

- Ovulation-Inducing Medications: For those trying to conceive, medications such as clomiphene citrate or letrozole can be prescribed to induce ovulation.

- Assisted Reproductive Techniques: In cases of severe ovulatory dysfunction, assisted reproductive techniques like in vitro fertilization (IVF) may be considered.

- Insulin-Sensitizing Drugs: Insulin-sensitizing medications can help improve ovulation by addressing insulin resistance.

- Regular Medical Monitoring: Regular check-ups and monitoring by healthcare professionals are crucial for tracking ovulation, hormone levels, and reproductive health.

Managing ovulatory dysfunction not only improves the chances of conception for those trying to become pregnant but also helps regulate menstrual cycles, alleviate symptoms, and reduce the risk of long-term complications associated with PCOS. It's important to work closely with healthcare providers to develop an individualized treatment plan based on specific needs and goals.

The ovarian cysts in PCOS

In Polycystic Ovary Syndrome (PCOS), the term "cysts" refers to small follicles (fluid-filled sacs) that develop on the ovaries. These follicles contain immature eggs that have not reached full maturity for ovulation. Despite the name "cysts," they are not the same as the larger, fluid-filled cysts that can develop in other conditions. Here's an explanation of the ovarian cysts in PCOS:

Characteristics of Ovarian Cysts in PCOS:

- In PCOS, the ovaries may contain numerous small follicles (cysts) that are typically less than 10 mm in diameter.
- These follicles are often arrested at an early stage of development and fail to mature and release an egg during ovulation. As a result, ovulation is disrupted or irregular.
- The hormonal imbalances present in PCOS contribute to the development of these follicles.

Visualizing Ovarian Cysts:
- These small follicles can be visualized using medical imaging techniques such as ultrasound.
- On ultrasound, the ovaries of individuals with PCOS may appear enlarged, with a "string of pearls" appearance, referring to the arrangement of multiple small cysts along the periphery of the ovary.

Relation to PCOS Diagnosis:
- The presence of these ovarian cysts is one of the criteria used for diagnosing PCOS, according to the Rotterdam criteria. However, it's important to note that not all individuals

with PCOS have visible ovarian cysts, and the presence of these cysts is not a mandatory requirement for diagnosis.

Impact on Ovulation:
- The presence of these small cysts contributes to ovulatory dysfunction in PCOS. The failure of these cysts to mature into ovulatory follicles results in irregular or absent ovulation.

Treatment:
- Addressing ovulatory dysfunction and hormonal imbalances are key aspects of managing PCOS.
- While the cysts themselves may not need to be treated directly, managing the underlying hormonal and metabolic factors can help regulate ovulation and improve fertility.

Monitoring and Management:
- Regular medical check-ups and monitoring by healthcare professionals are important for tracking ovarian health, hormonal levels, and overall well-being.

- Hormonal birth control and medications that induce ovulation can be used to manage the effects of the ovarian cysts and improve fertility.

Chapter 3: Unraveling the Causes

Genetic predisposition and hereditary factors

Genetic predisposition and hereditary factors play a significant role in the development of Polycystic Ovary Syndrome (PCOS). While the exact cause of PCOS is not fully understood, research indicates that both genetic and environmental factors contribute to its development. Here's an overview of how genetic predisposition and hereditary factors are linked to PCOS:

Genetic Predisposition:

- PCOS tends to run in families, suggesting a genetic component. If a close female family member (such as a mother, sister, or aunt) has PCOS, there is an increased likelihood of developing the condition.

Hereditary Factors:
- Several genes have been identified that may contribute to the development of PCOS. However, PCOS is a complex and multifactorial condition, meaning that it is influenced by interactions between multiple genes, rather than being caused by a single gene.
- These genetic factors can influence various aspects of PCOS, such as hormone regulation, insulin sensitivity, and ovarian function.

Insulin Signaling Pathways:
- Some of the genes implicated in PCOS are related to insulin signaling pathways. Insulin resistance is a common feature of PCOS, and genetic variations can impact how the body responds to insulin.
Androgen Metabolism:

- Genes involved in androgen metabolism and regulation can influence the production and metabolism of androgens (male hormones) in the body. Variations in these genes can contribute to the elevated androgen levels seen in PCOS.

Ovarian Function:
- Genetic factors can influence the development and function of the ovaries. Variations in genes related to follicular development and ovulation may contribute to the ovulatory dysfunction observed in PCOS.

Complex Interaction:
- It's important to note that while genetic predisposition plays a role, PCOS is a complex condition influenced by both genetic and environmental factors. Lifestyle choices, such as diet and physical activity, can interact with genetic predisposition to affect the severity and manifestation of PCOS symptoms.

Research and Understanding:

- Ongoing research is focused on identifying specific genes and genetic variations associated with PCOS. This knowledge can contribute to a better understanding of the condition's underlying mechanisms and potential targeted treatments.

Personalized Approach:
- Genetic predisposition is just one piece of the puzzle. Each individual's experience with PCOS is unique, and the interplay between genetic and environmental factors varies. Therefore, a personalized approach to diagnosis and management is essential.

While genetic predisposition and hereditary factors contribute to the development of PCOS, lifestyle changes, medical interventions, and ongoing healthcare support are crucial for managing the condition and its associated symptoms. Consulting with healthcare professionals can provide guidance tailored to individual needs and genetic predispositions.

Environmental influences and lifestyle correlations

Environmental influences and lifestyle factors play a significant role in the development and management of Polycystic Ovary Syndrome (PCOS). While genetic predisposition sets the stage, environmental factors can interact with genetics to influence the expression and severity of PCOS symptoms. Here's an overview of how environmental influences and lifestyle correlations impact PCOS:

1. Weight and Obesity:
- Excess body weight and obesity are associated with an increased risk of PCOS and can worsen its symptoms.
- Obesity contributes to insulin resistance, hormonal imbalances, and inflammation, all of which are characteristic features of PCOS.
- Losing even a modest amount of weight can improve insulin sensitivity, ovulation, and hormonal balance in women with PCOS.

2. Diet and Nutrition:

- Diet choices can influence insulin sensitivity and hormonal regulation. Consuming a diet high in refined carbohydrates and added sugars may contribute to insulin resistance.
- A balanced diet with a focus on whole foods, complex carbohydrates, lean proteins, and healthy fats can positively impact PCOS symptoms and overall health.

3. Physical Activity:
- Regular physical activity helps improve insulin sensitivity and can contribute to weight management.
- Exercise has been shown to positively influence menstrual regularity and reduce androgen levels in women with PCOS.

4. Stress and Mental Health:
- Chronic stress can impact hormonal balance and exacerbate PCOS symptoms. Stress management techniques, such as mindfulness and relaxation exercises, can be beneficial.
- PCOS-related symptoms, including changes in appearance and fertility struggles, can also contribute to emotional stress. Addressing

mental health is an important aspect of managing PCOS.

5. Sleep Quality:
- Poor sleep patterns and insufficient sleep have been linked to hormonal imbalances and insulin resistance.
- Prioritizing quality sleep can contribute to better overall health and hormonal regulation.

6. Environmental Exposures:
- Environmental factors, such as exposure to endocrine-disrupting chemicals, may play a role in hormonal imbalances and PCOS development.
- However, the exact impact of these factors on PCOS requires further research.

7. Lifestyle Modifications:
- Lifestyle modifications are a cornerstone of PCOS management. Adopting a healthier lifestyle can help improve insulin sensitivity, regulate menstrual cycles, and alleviate symptoms.

- Working with healthcare professionals to develop a personalized plan that includes dietary changes, exercise, stress management, and adequate sleep is crucial.

8. Ongoing Management:
- PCOS is a chronic condition that requires ongoing management. Maintaining a healthy lifestyle is essential for long-term symptom control and reducing the risk of associated health complications.

Understanding and addressing environmental influences and lifestyle factors are integral to managing PCOS effectively. A holistic approach that combines medical intervention with healthy habits can lead to improved quality of life and overall well-being for individuals with PCOS. Consulting with healthcare professionals can provide personalized guidance and support in making these lifestyle changes.

The complex interplay between genetics and environment

The development and manifestation of Polycystic Ovary Syndrome (PCOS) are influenced by a complex interplay between genetic factors and environmental influences. This interplay contributes to the variability in symptoms, severity, and outcomes observed among individuals with PCOS. Here's a deeper look into the intricate relationship between genetics and the environment in PCOS:

Genetic Predisposition:
- Genetic factors establish a predisposition for PCOS. Specific genes can influence hormone regulation, ovarian function, insulin sensitivity, and other aspects of the condition.
- A family history of PCOS increases the likelihood of developing the syndrome, suggesting a hereditary component.

Environmental Influences:
- Environmental factors interact with genetics to shape the expression and progression of PCOS. These factors include lifestyle, diet, stress, exposure to endocrine-disrupting chemicals, and more.

Complexity of Interaction:
- The interaction between genetics and the environment is complex and multifaceted. Genetic predisposition sets the stage, but environmental factors determine how PCOS develops and manifests.
- For example, individuals with a genetic predisposition to insulin resistance may experience worsened insulin sensitivity due to a sedentary lifestyle or poor dietary choices.

Epigenetics:
- Epigenetics refers to changes in gene expression that are influenced by environmental factors, without altering the underlying DNA sequence.
- Environmental factors such as nutrition, stress, and exposure to toxins can influence epigenetic changes that impact the development and progression of PCOS.

Variability in Symptoms:
- The interplay between genetics and the environment contributes to the variability in PCOS symptoms. Some individuals may have

more pronounced insulin resistance, while others may experience more severe androgen-related symptoms.

Lifestyle as a Modifier:
- Lifestyle choices can modify the impact of genetic predisposition. Adopting a healthy lifestyle, including balanced nutrition and regular exercise, can mitigate the effects of genetic risk factors and improve insulin sensitivity.

Personalized Approach:
- PCOS is not a one-size-fits-all condition. The unique genetic makeup of each individual interacts with their environment, resulting in diverse presentations of the syndrome.
- A personalized approach to diagnosis and management takes into account both genetic factors and environmental influences.

Research Implications:
- Research into the genetics of PCOS is ongoing, aiming to identify specific genes

and genetic variations associated with the condition.
- Understanding the interplay between genetics and environment is essential for developing targeted treatments and interventions.

In essence, PCOS arises from the intricate interplay between genetic predisposition and environmental influences. This complex relationship underscores the importance of personalized approaches to diagnosis, treatment, and lifestyle modifications for managing PCOS effectively.

Chapter 4: Diagnosis and Medical Assessment

Recognizing the symptoms and seeking medical help

Recognizing the symptoms of Polycystic Ovary Syndrome (PCOS) and seeking timely medical help is essential for early diagnosis, effective management, and prevention of potential complications. Here's a guide on recognizing PCOS symptoms and the importance of seeking medical assistance:

Common Symptoms of PCOS:
1. Irregular Menstrual Cycles: Irregular, infrequent, or absent periods are a hallmark of PCOS. Menstrual cycles may be longer or shorter than normal, or there may be months without a period.

2. Hirsutism: Excessive hair growth on the face, chest, back, or other areas where males typically grow hair is common in PCOS.

3. Acne and Oily Skin: Elevated androgen levels in PCOS can contribute to acne and oily skin.

4. Male-Pattern Baldness: Thinning hair or hair loss similar to male-pattern baldness can occur.

5. Weight Gain or Difficulty Losing Weight: PCOS is often associated with weight gain

and challenges in losing weight, especially around the abdomen.

6. Ovulatory Dysfunction: Infrequent or absent ovulation can lead to fertility issues and difficulty conceiving.

7. Insulin Resistance and Diabetes Risk: PCOS is linked to insulin resistance, increasing the risk of type 2 diabetes.

8. Mood Changes: Hormonal imbalances can contribute to mood swings, anxiety, and depression.

9. Skin Changes: Dark patches of skin (acanthosis nigricans) can develop in areas like the neck, armpits, or groin.

Seeking Medical Help:
1. Recognize Symptoms: Be aware of any changes or irregularities in your menstrual cycle, hair growth, skin health, and overall well-being.

2. Consult a Healthcare Professional: If you suspect you might have PCOS due to experiencing symptoms, schedule an appointment with a gynecologist, endocrinologist, or healthcare provider experienced in women's health.

3. Medical Evaluation: Your healthcare provider will perform a physical examination, review your medical history, and may order blood tests (hormone levels, glucose), ultrasound, and other tests to diagnose PCOS.

4. Early Diagnosis is Key: Early diagnosis allows for timely management and can help prevent potential complications such as diabetes, cardiovascular disease, and fertility issues.

5. Tailored Treatment Plan: Once diagnosed, your healthcare provider will work with you to develop a personalized treatment plan that may include lifestyle changes, medication, and ongoing medical monitoring.

6. Open Communication: Be open about your symptoms and concerns with your healthcare provider. Discuss your goals, whether they involve managing symptoms, improving fertility, or maintaining overall health.

Remember that PCOS is a manageable condition, and seeking medical help early can significantly improve your quality of life. Timely diagnosis and comprehensive management can help you address symptoms, reduce long-term health risks, and optimize your well-being.

Diagnostic criteria and tests used for PCOS diagnosis

The diagnosis of Polycystic Ovary Syndrome (PCOS) involves a combination of clinical assessment, medical history, physical examination, and specific tests. Various diagnostic criteria have been established to aid in identifying PCOS. The most commonly used criteria are those outlined by the Rotterdam criteria and the Androgen Excess and PCOS Society (AES) criteria. Here's an overview of the diagnostic criteria and tests used for PCOS diagnosis:

1. Rotterdam Criteria:
According to the Rotterdam criteria, a PCOS diagnosis can be made if at least two out of three following criteria are met:

1. Ovulatory Dysfunction: Irregular or absent menstrual cycles due to anovulation.
2. Clinical and/or Biochemical Signs of Hyperandrogenism: This includes hirsutism, acne, androgenic alopecia, or elevated androgen levels in blood tests.
3. Polycystic Ovaries: Presence of multiple small cysts on one or both ovaries, as visualized through ultrasound.

2. Androgen Excess and PCOS Society (AES) Criteria:
The AES criteria require the presence of hyperandrogenism (excessive androgens) and ovarian dysfunction (oligo-anovulation) for a PCOS diagnosis. Ovulatory dysfunction can be determined through clinical history or menstrual irregularities.

Diagnostic Tests:

- Blood Tests: Hormone level assessments, including measurements of androgens (testosterone, DHEAS), luteinizing hormone (LH), follicle-stimulating hormone (FSH), and insulin, can help identify hormonal imbalances associated with PCOS.

- Ultrasound: Transvaginal ultrasound is used to visualize the ovaries and identify the presence of multiple small cysts, known as follicles, in a characteristic pattern.

- Medical History and Physical Examination: Details about menstrual cycles, hirsutism, acne, and other symptoms are collected. A physical exam can reveal signs of hyperandrogenism, such as hirsutism and male-pattern hair loss.

- Glucose Tolerance Test: To assess insulin resistance and diabetes risk, a glucose tolerance test may be conducted.

Exclusion of Other Conditions:

Other conditions with similar symptoms, such as thyroid disorders and adrenal conditions, should be ruled out before a PCOS diagnosis is made.

Importance of Diagnosis:
An accurate diagnosis is crucial for tailored management. PCOS is a complex condition, and its symptoms can vary widely among individuals. With a proper diagnosis, healthcare professionals can create a personalized treatment plan that addresses specific symptoms and health risks.

If you suspect you have PCOS due to experiencing symptoms, it's important to consult a healthcare provider. Early diagnosis and proper management can lead to improved quality of life and better health outcomes.

Differential diagnoses and conditions to rule out

When diagnosing Polycystic Ovary Syndrome (PCOS), it's important for healthcare professionals to consider other conditions with similar symptoms. Proper differential diagnosis helps ensure accurate identification of the underlying issue and appropriate management. Here are some conditions that should be ruled out or considered during the diagnostic process:

1. Thyroid Disorders:
- Conditions like hypothyroidism or hyperthyroidism can cause irregular menstrual cycles, weight changes, fatigue, and mood disturbances similar to PCOS.

2. Hyperprolactinemia:
- Elevated levels of the hormone prolactin can lead to irregular periods, disrupted ovulation, and other symptoms resembling PCOS.

3. Non-Classical Congenital Adrenal Hyperplasia (NCAH):
- NCAH is a genetic disorder that can cause symptoms similar to PCOS, including androgen excess, irregular menstrual cycles, and hirsutism.

4. Cushing's Syndrome:
- Excessive production of cortisol, often due to adrenal tumors or prolonged steroid use, can lead to features resembling PCOS, such as weight gain, hirsutism, and irregular periods.

5. Ovarian Tumors:
- Ovarian tumors, such as androgen-secreting tumors, can cause androgen excess and menstrual irregularities similar to PCOS.

6. Adrenal Disorders:
- Conditions affecting the adrenal glands, such as congenital adrenal hyperplasia (CAH), can lead to androgen excess and symptoms resembling PCOS.

7. Hyperthecosis:
- Hyperthecosis involves the growth of ovarian tissue with excessive androgen production, leading to symptoms similar to PCOS.

8. Idiopathic Hirsutism:
- Some individuals may experience hirsutism without other PCOS symptoms. This condition is known as idiopathic hirsutism and requires differentiation from PCOS.

9. Premature Ovarian Insufficiency (POI):
- POI refers to the loss of ovarian function before the age of 40, leading to irregular periods and infertility. It can sometimes be mistaken for PCOS.

10. Adiposity-Related Conditions:
- Obesity itself can lead to hormonal imbalances, irregular periods, and insulin resistance, mimicking PCOS symptoms.

11. Pituitary Disorders:
- Conditions affecting the pituitary gland, such as pituitary tumors, can disrupt hormonal balance and lead to irregular periods and other symptoms resembling PCOS.

Proper diagnosis involves a thorough medical history, physical examination, and a range of tests, including blood work, hormonal assessments, ultrasound, and more. By ruling out other conditions and considering the complete clinical picture, healthcare professionals can accurately diagnose PCOS and provide appropriate treatment and management strategies. If you suspect you have PCOS or are experiencing symptoms, it's important to consult a qualified healthcare provider for an accurate assessment.

Importance of early detection and intervention

Early detection and intervention for Polycystic Ovary Syndrome (PCOS) are crucial for a variety of reasons, including better symptom management, improved quality of life, prevention of long-term health complications, and enhanced fertility outcomes. Here's why early detection and intervention matter:

1. Symptom Control:

- Early intervention allows for prompt management of PCOS symptoms, which can help improve overall well-being and prevent symptom progression.

2. Preventing Long-Term Health Risks:
- PCOS is associated with an increased risk of several long-term health issues, including type 2 diabetes, cardiovascular disease, and endometrial cancer.
- Early intervention can help mitigate these risks through lifestyle modifications, medication, and ongoing medical monitoring.

3. Fertility and Reproductive Health:
- Early diagnosis and treatment can improve fertility outcomes for individuals trying to conceive. Timely interventions can help regulate menstrual cycles, induce ovulation, and increase the chances of successful conception.

4. Psychological Well-Being:
- The physical symptoms of PCOS, along with the challenges of managing fertility and

hormonal imbalances, can impact mental health.
- Early intervention can address symptoms that contribute to psychological distress and improve overall emotional well-being.

5. Lifestyle Modifications:
- Early detection provides an opportunity to implement lifestyle modifications, such as adopting a balanced diet, increasing physical activity, and managing stress, which can improve insulin sensitivity and hormonal balance.

6. Customized Treatment Plans:
- Early diagnosis allows healthcare professionals to develop personalized treatment plans based on individual symptoms, needs, and goals.

7. Prevention of Unnecessary Interventions:
- Prompt diagnosis prevents unnecessary testing and interventions that may be prescribed when symptoms are left unaddressed.

8. Improved Patient Education:
- Early intervention allows individuals to better understand their condition, empowering them to make informed decisions about their health and treatment options.

9. Avoidance of Secondary Complications:
- Long-standing unmanaged PCOS can lead to complications like obesity, insulin resistance, and infertility. Early intervention can help prevent the development of these secondary complications.

10. Quality of Life Improvement:
- Timely intervention can greatly enhance the quality of life for individuals with PCOS by alleviating symptoms, improving self-esteem, and providing better control over their health.

Recognizing the symptoms of PCOS and seeking medical help early are the first steps towards effective management and prevention of potential complications. Consulting a healthcare provider, such as a gynecologist or endocrinologist, allows for accurate diagnosis, tailored treatment plans, and ongoing support to optimize physical and emotional well-being.

Chapter 5: Managing PCOS: Medical Approaches

Pharmacological treatments for symptom management

Pharmacological treatments play a significant role in managing the symptoms of Polycystic Ovary Syndrome (PCOS). These medications target specific aspects of the condition to alleviate symptoms, regulate hormonal imbalances, and improve overall well-being. Here's an overview of some common pharmacological treatments used for PCOS symptom management:

1. Hormonal Birth Control:
- Hormonal contraceptives, such as combination oral contraceptives (estrogen and progestin), can help regulate menstrual cycles and reduce androgen production,

leading to improvements in hirsutism, acne, and irregular periods.
- Birth control pills can also lower the risk of endometrial hyperplasia, which is a concern in PCOS due to irregular ovulation.

2. Anti-Androgen Medications:
- Anti-androgens, such as spironolactone and flutamide, help reduce the effects of elevated androgens. They can improve hirsutism, acne, and male-pattern hair loss.
- These medications work by blocking the action of androgens on target tissues.

3. Insulin-Sensitizing Medications:
- Insulin-sensitizing drugs like metformin help improve insulin sensitivity and can have positive effects on ovulation, menstrual regularity, and metabolic parameters.
- These medications are particularly useful for individuals with PCOS who also have insulin resistance.

4. Ovulation-Inducing Medications:
- Clomiphene citrate and letrozole are medications used to induce ovulation in women with PCOS who are trying to conceive.
- These medications can help regulate ovulation, increasing the chances of successful pregnancy.

5. Anti-Inflammatory Medications:
- In some cases, nonsteroidal anti-inflammatory drugs (NSAIDs) may be used to alleviate pelvic pain or discomfort associated with PCOS.

6. Hair Growth Inhibitors:
- Eflornithine cream is a topical medication that can slow down the growth of facial hair in women with hirsutism.

7. Fertility Treatments:
- For individuals struggling with fertility due to anovulation, assisted reproductive techniques such as in vitro fertilization (IVF) can be considered.

8. Psychological Support and Antidepressants:
- Managing the psychological impact of PCOS is important. If mood disturbances or anxiety are significant, mental health support and, in some cases, antidepressant medications may be recommended.

Individualized Approach:
- Treatment plans should be individualized based on symptoms, patient preferences, and health goals.
- The severity of symptoms and the desire for pregnancy are important factors in determining the appropriate pharmacological approach.

Consulting with a healthcare provider, such as a gynecologist or endocrinologist, is crucial before starting any pharmacological treatment. Healthcare professionals will assess your medical history, symptoms, and health goals to determine the most appropriate medication or combination of medications for your unique situation.

Hormonal birth control options and their benefits

Hormonal birth control options offer a range of benefits for individuals with Polycystic Ovary Syndrome (PCOS). These methods can help regulate menstrual cycles, manage hormonal imbalances, and alleviate symptoms associated with PCOS. Here are some common hormonal birth control options and their benefits for PCOS symptom management:

1. Combination Oral Contraceptives (COCs):
- COCs contain both estrogen and progestin hormones.
- Benefits: COCs can regulate menstrual cycles, reduce androgen production, improve hirsutism and acne, and lower the risk of endometrial hyperplasia.
- Considerations: They are contraindicated in women with certain medical conditions, such as a history of blood clots, smoking, or certain cardiovascular conditions.

2. Progestin-Only Pills (Mini Pills):

- Mini pills contain only progestin.
- Benefits: Progestin-only pills can help regulate menstrual cycles and provide birth control options for individuals who cannot tolerate estrogen.
- Considerations: They need to be taken consistently at the same time each day for maximum effectiveness.

3. Hormonal Patch:

- The patch delivers estrogen and progestin through the skin.
- Benefits: It provides continuous hormonal regulation similar to COCs, but with a weekly patch application.
- Considerations: The patch needs to be applied and replaced weekly.

4. Hormonal Ring:

- The vaginal ring releases estrogen and progestin.
- Benefits: Similar to COCs, the ring provides hormonal regulation with a monthly application.

- Considerations: It needs to be inserted and replaced monthly.

5. Hormonal Intrauterine Device (IUD):
- Hormonal IUDs, such as the Mirena, release progestin locally into the uterus.
- Benefits: They can reduce menstrual bleeding and regulate cycles. Some individuals may experience a decrease in hirsutism and acne.
- Considerations: IUD insertion requires a healthcare provider and may cause discomfort initially.

6. Continuous or Extended Cycle COCs:
- These are COCs taken continuously to suppress menstruation.
- Benefits: They can help manage heavy bleeding and regulate cycles while minimizing the number of periods experienced.

Benefits of Hormonal Birth Control for PCOS:
- Regulation of Menstrual Cycles: Hormonal birth control can help establish regular, predictable menstrual cycles.
- Hormonal Imbalance Management: Birth control methods can reduce androgens, which helps manage hirsutism, acne, and male-pattern hair loss.
- Lower Risk of Endometrial Hyperplasia: Regular use of hormonal birth control can reduce the risk of overgrowth of the uterine lining.
- Enhanced Quality of Life: Alleviating PCOS symptoms can lead to improved emotional well-being and self-esteem.

Individual preferences, health considerations, and lifestyle factors should guide the choice of hormonal birth control. Consulting a healthcare provider is crucial to select the most suitable option based on your unique needs and goals.

Insulin-sensitizing medications and their role

Insulin-sensitizing medications are a class of drugs used to improve insulin sensitivity in individuals with conditions such as Polycystic Ovary Syndrome (PCOS) or type 2 diabetes. These medications can play a significant role in managing PCOS by addressing insulin resistance, which is a common feature of the condition. Here are some commonly used insulin-sensitizing medications and their role in PCOS management:

1. Metformin:
- Metformin is the most commonly prescribed insulin-sensitizing medication for PCOS.
- Mechanism of Action: Metformin reduces glucose production in the liver, enhances insulin sensitivity in muscle tissue, and improves the uptake of glucose by cells.
- Benefits: Metformin helps lower blood glucose levels, improve insulin sensitivity, and regulate menstrual cycles in women with PCOS. It can also contribute to weight loss and reduction of androgen levels.
- Considerations: Side effects may include gastrointestinal symptoms, such as nausea

and diarrhea, but these often improve over time. Metformin is generally well-tolerated.

2. Thiazolidinediones (TZDs):
- Thiazolidinediones, such as pioglitazone, are another class of insulin-sensitizing medications.
- Mechanism of Action: TZDs work by increasing insulin sensitivity in peripheral tissues, such as muscle and fat cells.
- Benefits: TZDs can improve insulin resistance and may have positive effects on ovulation, menstrual regularity, and lipid profiles. However, they are less commonly used due to potential side effects and safety concerns.

3. Inositol:
- Inositol is a natural supplement that can function as an insulin-sensitizing agent.
- Mechanism of Action: Inositol is involved in insulin signaling pathways and can improve insulin sensitivity.
- Benefits: Some studies suggest that inositol supplementation may help regulate menstrual

cycles, improve fertility, and reduce insulin resistance in women with PCOS.

4. Lifestyle Modifications:
- While not medications, lifestyle modifications such as adopting a healthy diet and increasing physical activity can also improve insulin sensitivity.

Role of Insulin-Sensitizing Medications in PCOS:
- Regulating Insulin Resistance: Insulin-sensitizing medications primarily address insulin resistance, which is a common underlying factor in PCOS.
- Improving Ovulation and Menstrual Regularity: By enhancing insulin sensitivity, these medications can help regulate menstrual cycles and promote ovulation.
- Managing Metabolic Health: Insulin-sensitizing medications can improve glucose control and reduce the risk of type 2 diabetes in individuals with PCOS.
- Addressing Androgen Excess: Some insulin-sensitizing medications may help

reduce androgen levels, leading to improvements in hirsutism and acne.

It's important to note that individual response to insulin-sensitizing medications can vary. Healthcare providers assess factors such as medical history, overall health, and treatment goals when determining the appropriate medication and dosage for each individual. Lifestyle modifications, in combination with medications, can provide a comprehensive approach to managing insulin resistance and improving overall well-being for individuals with PCOS.

Managing infertility and assisted reproductive techniques

Managing infertility in individuals with Polycystic Ovary Syndrome (PCOS) often involves a combination of lifestyle modifications, medication, and assisted reproductive techniques. PCOS-related infertility is primarily due to anovulation (lack of ovulation) or irregular ovulation.

Here's an overview of how infertility associated with PCOS can be managed:

1. Lifestyle Modifications:
- Weight Management: Achieving and maintaining a healthy weight can improve hormonal balance, enhance ovulation, and increase the chances of conception.
- Balanced Diet: Adopting a balanced diet with complex carbohydrates, lean proteins, healthy fats, and fiber can support hormonal regulation and fertility.
- Physical Activity: Regular exercise can help improve insulin sensitivity, promote weight loss, and contribute to overall reproductive health.

2. Medications:
- Ovulation-Inducing Medications: Clomiphene citrate and letrozole are commonly used medications to induce ovulation in individuals with PCOS. They help stimulate follicle development and improve the chances of successful conception.

- Gonadotropins: If ovulation induction medications are not effective, gonadotropin injections can be used to stimulate multiple follicles to develop.

3. Assisted Reproductive Techniques (ART):
- Intrauterine Insemination (IUI): IUI involves placing washed sperm directly into the uterus during ovulation. This can improve the chances of sperm reaching and fertilizing the egg.
- In Vitro Fertilization (IVF): IVF is a more advanced technique where eggs are retrieved, fertilized in a laboratory, and then transferred back into the uterus.
- Ovarian Hyperstimulation: In some cases, controlled ovarian hyperstimulation is used to develop multiple follicles, increasing the chances of successful IVF.

4. Oocyte (Egg) Freezing:
- For individuals with PCOS who may experience irregular ovulation, egg freezing

can be considered to preserve fertility options for the future.

5. Hormonal Support:
- Hormonal support during fertility treatments may involve medications to enhance endometrial lining growth and support early pregnancy.

6. Psychological Support:
- Infertility can be emotionally challenging. Seeking counseling or support groups can help manage the psychological aspects of fertility treatments.

7. Individualized Approach:
- Fertility treatments are highly individualized and should be tailored to each person's needs, preferences, and medical history.

8. Monitoring and Follow-Up:
- Close monitoring by fertility specialists is crucial to track ovulation, adjust medication dosages, and ensure timely interventions.

Remember that success rates for fertility treatments can vary based on factors such as age, health status, and treatment history. Consultation with a reproductive endocrinologist or fertility specialist is essential to develop a personalized fertility plan that addresses your specific circumstances and goals. With the right approach and medical guidance, many individuals with PCOS can successfully achieve pregnancy and expand their families.

Chapter 6: Lifestyle Modifications and Self-Care

The impact of diet and nutrition on PCOS

Diet and nutrition play a significant role in the management of Polycystic Ovary Syndrome (PCOS). Making healthy dietary choices can help regulate hormonal imbalances, improve insulin sensitivity, manage weight, and alleviate PCOS-related symptoms. Here's how diet and nutrition can impact PCOS:

1. Insulin Sensitivity:

- PCOS is often associated with insulin resistance, which can lead to elevated blood sugar levels and hormonal imbalances.
- A diet focused on complex carbohydrates, fiber-rich foods, and balanced meals can help improve insulin sensitivity and regulate blood sugar levels.

2. Weight Management:
- Maintaining a healthy weight can positively influence hormonal balance and fertility outcomes for individuals with PCOS.
- A balanced diet that controls calorie intake and includes nutrient-dense foods can support weight management goals.

3. Carbohydrate Choices:
- Choosing complex carbohydrates, such as whole grains, legumes, vegetables, and fruits, can help prevent rapid spikes in blood sugar and insulin levels.

4. Protein Intake:

- Including lean protein sources, such as poultry, fish, beans, and tofu, can help stabilize blood sugar levels and support muscle health.

5. Healthy Fats:
- Consuming sources of healthy fats, like avocados, nuts, seeds, and olive oil, can contribute to satiety and help maintain steady energy levels.

6. Omega-3 Fatty Acids:
- Omega-3 fatty acids, found in fatty fish (salmon, mackerel) and flaxseeds, have anti-inflammatory properties that can benefit individuals with PCOS.

7. Dairy and Calcium:
- Including low-fat or non-fat dairy products and calcium-rich foods can support bone health and provide essential nutrients.

8. Anti-Inflammatory Foods:
- Incorporating foods rich in antioxidants and anti-inflammatory compounds, such as

colorful fruits and vegetables, can help
manage inflammation associated with PCOS.

9. Fiber-Rich Foods:
- High-fiber foods like whole grains, fruits,
vegetables, and legumes can promote
digestive health, aid in weight management,
and stabilize blood sugar levels.

10. Nutrient Supplementation:
- Some individuals with PCOS may benefit
from specific nutrient supplementation, such
as inositol, which can help improve insulin
sensitivity.

11. Hydration:
- Drinking plenty of water is essential for
overall health and can support metabolic
processes and hormone regulation.

12. Portion Control and Mindful Eating:
- Paying attention to portion sizes and
practicing mindful eating can prevent

overeating and promote a healthy relationship with food.

13. Limit Processed Foods and Sugars:
- Minimizing processed foods, sugary snacks, and sugary beverages can help regulate blood sugar levels and prevent insulin spikes.

A registered dietitian or nutritionist with experience in PCOS can provide personalized guidance on creating a diet plan that suits your needs and goals. A balanced diet, combined with regular physical activity and other lifestyle modifications, forms the foundation for effectively managing PCOS and improving overall well-being.

Exercise and physical activity recommendations

Exercise and physical activity are important components of managing Polycystic Ovary Syndrome (PCOS). Regular exercise can help improve insulin sensitivity, regulate hormonal imbalances, support weight management, and enhance overall well-being. Here are some exercise and physical activity recommendations for individuals with PCOS:

1. Aerobic Exercise:
- Aim for at least 150 minutes of moderate-intensity aerobic exercise per week, spread out over several days.
- Activities like brisk walking, jogging, cycling, swimming, and dancing can help improve cardiovascular health and contribute to weight management.

2. Strength Training:
- Incorporate strength training exercises at least two days a week.
- Strength training with weights, resistance bands, or bodyweight exercises can help build muscle mass, boost metabolism, and improve insulin sensitivity.

3. High-Intensity Interval Training (HIIT):
- HIIT involves alternating between short bursts of intense exercise and lower-intensity recovery periods.

- HIIT workouts can be effective for improving cardiovascular fitness and burning calories in a shorter amount of time.

4. Flexibility and Stretching:
- Include flexibility exercises or stretching in your routine to improve joint mobility and prevent muscle tightness.

5. Balance and Core Exercises:
- Integrating exercises that target balance and core stability can improve posture and prevent injuries.

6. Physical Activities You Enjoy:
- Engage in activities you enjoy, whether it's dancing, hiking, yoga, or playing a sport. Enjoyable activities are more likely to be sustained long-term.

7. Consistency:
- Aim for regular physical activity. Consistency is key to reaping the benefits of exercise.

8. Gradual Progression:
- Start at a level that's comfortable for you and gradually increase intensity, duration, or frequency over time.

9. Consult a Healthcare Professional:
- If you're new to exercise or have any health concerns, consult a healthcare provider before starting a new exercise routine.

10. Tailored Approach:
- Consider working with a fitness professional, such as a personal trainer or exercise physiologist, to develop a personalized exercise plan that aligns with your goals and needs.

11. Lifestyle Integration:
- Look for opportunities to increase physical activity in your daily life, such as taking the stairs instead of the elevator, walking more, or engaging in active hobbies.

12. Listen to Your Body:

- Pay attention to your body's signals. If you experience pain, fatigue, or discomfort, adjust your exercise intensity or seek medical advice.

Exercise should be part of a comprehensive approach that includes a balanced diet, proper hydration, adequate sleep, and stress management. Engaging in regular physical activity can contribute to better PCOS management, improved mood, and enhanced overall health.

Stress management techniques and their significance

Stress management techniques are essential for individuals with Polycystic Ovary Syndrome (PCOS) to improve overall well-being and effectively manage the condition. Chronic stress can exacerbate PCOS symptoms and hormonal imbalances, making stress management a crucial aspect of a comprehensive approach to PCOS care. Here's why stress management is significant and some techniques to consider:

Significance of Stress Management:
1. Hormonal Balance: Chronic stress can disrupt hormonal balance and exacerbate PCOS-related symptoms, such as irregular periods, acne, and hirsutism.
2. Insulin Sensitivity: Stress hormones can impact insulin sensitivity, aggravating insulin resistance, a common feature of PCOS.
3. Weight Management: Stress can contribute to emotional eating and weight gain, which can worsen PCOS symptoms and insulin resistance.
4. Inflammation: Stress triggers an inflammatory response in the body, which can contribute to various health issues, including PCOS-related inflammation.
5. Fertility: Stress can impact reproductive health and fertility outcomes.

Stress Management Techniques:
1. Mindfulness Meditation: Practicing mindfulness can help you stay present and reduce stress. Techniques include deep breathing, body scans, and guided meditation.

2. Yoga: Yoga combines physical movement, breathing exercises, and relaxation techniques to reduce stress and promote well-being.

3. Exercise: Regular physical activity can reduce stress hormones and boost mood through the release of endorphins.

4. Journaling: Writing down your thoughts and feelings can help you process emotions and gain insights into sources of stress.

5. Social Support: Connecting with friends, family, or support groups can provide emotional outlets and reduce feelings of isolation.

6. Time Management: Organize tasks, prioritize responsibilities, and allocate time for self-care to reduce feelings of overwhelm.

7. Progressive Muscle Relaxation: Tension and relaxation exercises can help relieve physical and mental tension caused by stress.

8. Deep Breathing: Deep, slow breathing can activate the body's relaxation response and reduce stress.

9. Hobbies and Activities: Engaging in activities you enjoy, whether it's reading, crafting, or gardening, can be a form of stress relief.

10. Limiting Stressors: Identify sources of stress in your life and make efforts to reduce or eliminate them where possible.

11. Professional Help: If stress becomes overwhelming, seeking help from a therapist or counselor can provide effective coping strategies.

Remember that stress management is a continuous practice. Finding the techniques that work best for you and integrating them into your daily routine can lead to improved PCOS management, better emotional well-being, and overall enhanced quality of life.

Importance of sleep and maintaining a healthy routine

Sleep and maintaining a healthy routine are critical components of managing Polycystic Ovary Syndrome (PCOS) and promoting overall well-being. Both sleep quality and a balanced daily routine play significant roles in hormonal balance, metabolic health, stress management, and symptom control. Here's why sleep and a healthy routine are important for individuals with PCOS:

Importance of Sleep:
1. Hormonal Regulation: Adequate sleep supports the proper functioning of hormonal systems, including those related to insulin, cortisol, and reproductive hormones.
2. Insulin Sensitivity: Poor sleep can disrupt insulin sensitivity, contributing to insulin resistance, which is common in PCOS.
3. Metabolic Health: Sleep deprivation is associated with weight gain, which can worsen PCOS symptoms and insulin resistance.
4. Stress Reduction: Quality sleep helps manage stress levels and prevents the release of stress hormones that can worsen PCOS symptoms.
5. Reproductive Health: Sleep supports the regulation of reproductive hormones, menstrual cycles, and ovulation.

Importance of a Healthy Routine:

1. Stable Blood Sugar Levels: Consistent meal timing and balanced meals can help stabilize blood sugar levels and manage insulin resistance.

2. Weight Management: A routine that includes regular exercise and mindful eating can support weight management, which is important for PCOS.

3. Hormonal Balance: A healthy routine contributes to hormonal balance, reducing the severity of PCOS-related symptoms.

4. Stress Management: A structured routine with time for relaxation and self-care can mitigate the impact of chronic stress.

5. Consistent Habits: A routine can promote healthy habits, making it easier to manage PCOS symptoms in the long term.

Tips for Improving Sleep and Maintaining a Healthy Routine:

1. Prioritize Sleep: Aim for 7-9 hours of quality sleep each night. Create a calming bedtime routine and ensure a comfortable sleep environment.

2. Consistent Wake Time: Wake up at the same time every day to regulate your body's internal clock.

3. Regular Meals: Eat balanced meals and snacks at regular intervals to stabilize blood sugar levels.

4. Hydration: Drink plenty of water throughout the day to stay hydrated.

5. Physical Activity: Incorporate regular exercise into your routine, but avoid vigorous exercise close to bedtime.

6. Mindful Eating: Pay attention to hunger and fullness cues while eating. Avoid large, heavy meals before bedtime.

7. Stress Reduction: Dedicate time to relaxation techniques such as meditation, deep breathing, or yoga.

8. Limit Caffeine and Screens: Limit caffeine intake in the afternoon and avoid screens (phones, computers) before bedtime.

9. Social Time: Maintain connections with friends and family, which can provide emotional support and reduce stress.

10. Stay Consistent: Stick to your routine as much as possible, even on weekends.

By prioritizing sleep and establishing a healthy routine, individuals with PCOS can optimize hormonal balance, metabolic health, stress management, and overall well-being. Consult with healthcare professionals for personalized guidance tailored to your unique needs and goals.

Chapter 7: Fertility and Pregnancy with PCOS

Understanding ovulation and optimizing chances of conception

Understanding ovulation and optimizing chances of conception is crucial for individuals with Polycystic Ovary Syndrome (PCOS) who are trying to get pregnant. PCOS can affect ovulation, making it important to track ovulation and use strategies to increase the likelihood of successful conception. Here's what you need to know:

Ovulation and PCOS:
- Ovulation is the release of an egg from the ovaries, allowing for the possibility of fertilization by sperm.
- PCOS is often associated with anovulation (lack of ovulation) or irregular ovulation, which can impact fertility.

Tracking Ovulation:

- Monitoring your menstrual cycle is key. While cycles can be irregular in PCOS, tracking can help identify patterns.
- Tools such as ovulation predictor kits (OPKs), basal body temperature (BBT) charting, and cervical mucus monitoring can assist in predicting ovulation.

Optimizing Chances of Conception:
1. Lifestyle Modifications: Adopt a healthy lifestyle with balanced nutrition, regular exercise, and stress management. A healthy weight can enhance fertility.
2. Consult a Healthcare Provider: Seek guidance from a healthcare provider, such as a reproductive endocrinologist or OB/GYN, who specializes in fertility and PCOS.
3. Ovulation-Inducing Medications: If you're not ovulating regularly, your doctor may prescribe medications like clomiphene citrate or letrozole to induce ovulation.
4. Regular Intercourse: Aim for regular sexual intercourse throughout your cycle, with a focus on the days around ovulation.

5. Ovulation Prediction: Use OPKs or other tracking methods to predict ovulation and time intercourse accordingly.
6. Basal Body Temperature (BBT) Charting: Track your basal body temperature daily to detect a rise, which indicates ovulation.
7. Cervical Mucus Changes: Monitor changes in cervical mucus consistency, which becomes clear and slippery around ovulation.
8. Health Check: Ensure that you and your partner are in good health, addressing any underlying medical conditions.
9. Patience: Conception might take time, so be patient and persistent. Seek support from loved ones and professionals.
10. Stress Reduction: Manage stress through relaxation techniques, exercise, and mindfulness. High stress levels can affect fertility.

Seeking Fertility Specialist Help:
If you've been trying to conceive for a while without success, it's advisable to consult a fertility specialist. They can perform thorough assessments, recommend

appropriate tests, and tailor interventions to your specific situation.

Remember that every individual's journey to conception is unique. Tracking ovulation and implementing strategies to optimize your chances, along with professional guidance, can increase the likelihood of achieving a successful pregnancy.

PCOS-related challenges in pregnancy

Pregnancy for individuals with Polycystic Ovary Syndrome (PCOS) can present certain challenges due to the hormonal imbalances and metabolic issues associated with the condition. While many women with PCOS have healthy pregnancies, it's important to be aware of potential challenges and work closely with healthcare providers to ensure a safe and successful pregnancy. Here are some PCOS-related challenges that may arise during pregnancy:

1. Gestational Diabetes:

- Women with PCOS have a higher risk of developing gestational diabetes, a type of diabetes that occurs during pregnancy.
- Close monitoring of blood sugar levels and dietary adjustments may be necessary to manage gestational diabetes.

2. Insulin Resistance:
- Insulin resistance, common in PCOS, can persist during pregnancy and increase the risk of gestational diabetes.
- Managing insulin resistance through diet, exercise, and possibly medication is important.

3. Hypertension (High Blood Pressure):
- PCOS is associated with an increased risk of developing high blood pressure during pregnancy, a condition known as gestational hypertension.
- Regular blood pressure monitoring and medical management are essential to prevent complications.
4. Preterm Birth and Preeclampsia:
- Women with PCOS may have a slightly increased risk of preterm birth and

preeclampsia (high blood pressure and organ damage during pregnancy).
- Regular prenatal care, monitoring, and management are crucial to reduce these risks.

5. Increased Risk of Cesarean Section:
- Women with PCOS may have a higher likelihood of delivering by cesarean section due to factors such as gestational diabetes and larger babies.

6. Monitoring Baby's Growth:
- Some women with PCOS may have larger babies (macrosomia) due to insulin resistance.
- Regular ultrasounds and monitoring of baby's growth are important.

7. Emotional Health:
- The hormonal and emotional challenges associated with PCOS can impact mental well-being during pregnancy.
- Seeking support from healthcare providers, counselors, and support groups can help manage emotional health.

8. Postpartum Concerns:
- Hormonal imbalances and insulin resistance can persist postpartum, potentially affecting recovery and lactation.
- Managing health postpartum through proper medical care, diet, and exercise is important.

9. Lifestyle Management:
- Continued focus on a healthy lifestyle, including diet and exercise, is essential during pregnancy to manage PCOS-related challenges.

10. Healthcare Provider Collaboration:
- Regular communication and collaboration with an OB/GYN and other healthcare providers experienced in managing PCOS during pregnancy are crucial.

Each pregnancy is unique, and the challenges faced can vary. Open communication with healthcare providers, adherence to prenatal care, and a proactive approach to managing

PCOS-related challenges can help ensure a healthy and successful pregnancy outcome.

Managing gestational diabetes and other complications

Managing gestational diabetes and other complications during pregnancy, especially for individuals with Polycystic Ovary Syndrome (PCOS), requires close collaboration with healthcare providers and adherence to recommended strategies. Here are some guidelines for managing gestational diabetes and other potential complications:

1. Gestational Diabetes Management:
- Regular Monitoring: Monitor blood sugar levels as advised by your healthcare provider. Keeping blood sugar within target ranges is essential.
- Balanced Diet: Follow a balanced diet recommended by a registered dietitian or healthcare provider. Focus on complex carbohydrates, lean proteins, and healthy fats.
- Portion Control: Control portion sizes to avoid spikes in blood sugar levels.

- Regular Meals: Eat regular, balanced meals and avoid skipping meals.
- Physical Activity: Engage in regular, safe physical activity as recommended by your healthcare provider. Exercise can help regulate blood sugar levels.
- Medication (if needed): In some cases, insulin or other medications may be prescribed to manage blood sugar levels.
- Fetal Monitoring: Your healthcare provider will closely monitor the baby's growth and development through regular ultrasounds.

2. Blood Pressure Management:
- Regular Monitoring: Monitor blood pressure at home as advised by your healthcare provider.
- Sodium Intake: Limit sodium intake to help manage blood pressure.
- Physical Activity: Engage in safe, moderate physical activity to support healthy blood pressure.

3. Preeclampsia Prevention:

- Regular Prenatal Visits: Attend all prenatal appointments to monitor blood pressure and other indicators of preeclampsia.
- Blood Pressure Management: Follow recommendations from your healthcare provider to manage blood pressure.
- Monitoring Symptoms: Be aware of symptoms like severe headaches, vision changes, and swelling, and report them to your healthcare provider.

4. Emotional Well-being:
- Seek Support: Share any emotional concerns with your healthcare provider and consider joining support groups for individuals with PCOS and gestational diabetes.
- Stress Reduction: Practice stress reduction techniques, such as meditation, deep breathing, and gentle exercise.

5. Postpartum Care:

- Continue Monitoring: Regular postpartum check-ups are important to monitor blood sugar levels and overall health.
- Lactation: If breastfeeding, continue managing blood sugar levels and follow a balanced diet to support lactation.

6. Healthcare Provider Collaboration:
- Maintain regular communication with your OB/GYN, endocrinologist, and other healthcare providers to ensure a coordinated approach to managing your health.

7. Lifestyle Factors:
- Focus on a healthy lifestyle, including a balanced diet, regular exercise, stress management, and adequate sleep.

Remember: Every pregnancy is unique. The recommendations and strategies may vary based on individual circumstances. Adhering to medical advice, attending all recommended appointments, and collaborating closely with healthcare providers can help manage complications and ensure a safe and healthy pregnancy.

Postpartum considerations and long-term health planning

Postpartum considerations and long-term health planning are important aspects for individuals with Polycystic Ovary Syndrome (PCOS) who have recently given birth. Managing your health postpartum and planning for the long term can help you maintain well-being, manage PCOS symptoms, and reduce the risk of future complications. Here are some key points to consider:

Postpartum Considerations:
1. Hormonal Changes: Be prepared for hormonal fluctuations postpartum, which can impact mood and energy levels. Seek support from healthcare providers and loved ones if needed.
2. Breastfeeding: If breastfeeding, maintaining a balanced diet and managing blood sugar levels is crucial to support lactation and postpartum recovery.

3. Physical Recovery: Allow yourself time to recover physically after childbirth. Focus on gentle movements and exercises recommended by your healthcare provider.

4. Continued Blood Sugar Monitoring: If you had gestational diabetes, continue monitoring blood sugar levels postpartum as advised by your healthcare provider.

5. Emotional Well-being: Address any postpartum mood changes, such as postpartum depression or anxiety, with the help of healthcare professionals.

6. Support System: Surround yourself with a strong support system, including healthcare providers, family, and friends, to assist in your postpartum journey.

Long-Term Health Planning:

1. PCOS Management: Continue managing PCOS through a healthy lifestyle, including balanced nutrition, regular exercise, stress management, and adequate sleep.

2. Regular Check-ups: Schedule regular check-ups with your healthcare provider to monitor hormonal balance, blood sugar levels, and overall health.

3. Contraception: Discuss contraception options with your healthcare provider to prevent unplanned pregnancies if desired.

4. Weight Management: Focus on maintaining a healthy weight through diet and exercise to manage PCOS symptoms and reduce the risk of complications.

5. Future Fertility: If you plan to have more children in the future, discuss fertility considerations with your healthcare provider and consider long-term health planning.

6. Cardiovascular Health: Pay attention to heart health and risk factors for cardiovascular disease, which may be elevated in individuals with PCOS.

7. Regular Blood Sugar Monitoring: Maintain awareness of blood sugar levels, especially if you had gestational diabetes, and work with your healthcare provider to manage them.

Remember: Postpartum and long-term health planning should be personalized based on your individual circumstances, preferences, and goals. Consult your healthcare provider to create a comprehensive plan that addresses

your specific needs and ensures a healthy
future for you and your family.

Chapter 8: Emotional Well-being and PCOS

Addressing the emotional impact of PCOS

Addressing the emotional impact of
Polycystic Ovary Syndrome (PCOS) is
crucial, as the condition can have significant
psychological and emotional effects on
individuals. Managing the emotional aspects
of PCOS is an integral part of holistic care.

Here are some strategies to help address the emotional impact of PCOS:

1. Education and Understanding:
- Learn about PCOS to better understand the condition, its symptoms, and its potential effects on emotional well-being.
- Understanding the underlying causes and how they relate to hormonal and metabolic changes can help reduce feelings of confusion or self-blame.

2. Seek Professional Support:
- Consult a mental health professional, such as a therapist or counselor, who has experience in dealing with PCOS-related emotional challenges.
- Therapists can provide coping strategies, support, and a safe space to discuss emotions and concerns.

3. Support Networks:
- Connect with support groups, online forums, or local communities of individuals with PCOS. Sharing experiences and advice

with others can help reduce feelings of isolation.

4. Self-Care:
- Prioritize self-care activities that promote relaxation and well-being, such as meditation, deep breathing, yoga, or mindfulness.
- Engage in activities you enjoy to help manage stress and boost your mood.

5. Balanced Lifestyle:
- Adopt a balanced lifestyle that includes regular exercise, a nutritious diet, and sufficient sleep. These factors can positively impact emotional well-being.

6. Communication:
- Openly communicate with loved ones, friends, and partners about your experiences, emotions, and needs.
- Sharing your feelings can help them better understand what you're going through and offer support.

7. Set Realistic Goals:

- Set achievable goals for managing PCOS
symptoms and emotional challenges.
Celebrate small victories along the way.

8. Positive Self-Talk:
- Practice positive self-talk and challenge
negative thoughts. Replace self-criticism with
self-compassion and self-acceptance.

9. Professional Help for Fertility Concerns:
- If fertility concerns are causing emotional
distress, consult a fertility specialist who can
provide guidance and potential treatment
options.

10. Medication and Treatment:
- In some cases, individuals with PCOS may
experience mood disorders. If needed, discuss
medication or therapy options with a
healthcare provider.

11. Patience:
- Remember that managing emotions and
adapting to life with PCOS is a journey. Be

patient with yourself and acknowledge that it's okay to have both good and difficult days.

Addressing the emotional impact of PCOS requires a holistic approach that considers both physical and mental well-being. Each individual's experience is unique, so finding strategies that resonate with you and seeking professional support when needed can help you navigate the emotional challenges of PCOS more effectively.

Coping strategies for dealing with stress and anxiety

Dealing with stress and anxiety, whether related to Polycystic Ovary Syndrome (PCOS) or other life factors, requires a combination of coping strategies to help manage and alleviate these feelings. Here are some effective coping strategies that you can consider:

1. Deep Breathing and Relaxation:

- Practice deep breathing exercises to calm your nervous system and reduce stress. Techniques like diaphragmatic breathing or the 4-7-8 method can be helpful.
- Progressive muscle relaxation and guided imagery can also induce relaxation.

2. Mindfulness and Meditation:
- Engage in mindfulness meditation to stay present and reduce anxiety about the past or future.
- Mindfulness can be practiced through meditation, focusing on your breath, or being fully present in the moment.

3. Exercise and Physical Activity:
- Regular physical activity can release endorphins, which are natural mood elevators.
- Activities like walking, jogging, yoga, or dancing can help reduce stress and anxiety.

4. Healthy Lifestyle:

- Prioritize a balanced diet, adequate sleep, and regular exercise to support overall well-being and resilience against stress.

5. Time Management:
- Organize your tasks and responsibilities to prevent feeling overwhelmed. Prioritize and break tasks into smaller, manageable steps.

6. Journaling:
- Write down your thoughts and feelings to gain perspective on what's causing stress and anxiety.
- Journaling can provide an outlet for emotions and help identify patterns or triggers.

7. Social Support:
- Connect with friends, family, or support groups. Talking about your feelings and receiving empathy can alleviate stress.

8. Creative Outlets:
- Engage in creative activities you enjoy, such as drawing, painting, writing, or playing a musical instrument.

9. Limiting Stressors:
- Identify stressors in your life and consider ways to minimize or eliminate them where possible.

10. Set Realistic Goals:
- Break down your goals into achievable steps. Setting small, realistic goals can reduce feelings of pressure and anxiety.

11. Seek Professional Help:
- If stress and anxiety are interfering with your daily life, consider consulting a mental health professional for guidance and support.

12. Positive Self-Talk:
- Challenge negative thoughts and replace them with positive affirmations. Practice self-compassion and self-acceptance.

13. Limiting Stimulants:
- Reduce or limit caffeine intake, as excessive caffeine can contribute to feelings of jitteriness and anxiety.

14. Laughter and Humor:
- Engage in activities that make you laugh, watch a funny movie, or spend time with people who bring joy to your life.

15. Practice Gratitude:
- Focus on the positive aspects of your life. Practicing gratitude can shift your perspective and reduce anxiety.

Remember that everyone is different, so it may take some trial and error to find the coping strategies that work best for you. Combining multiple strategies and seeking professional support when needed can contribute to effectively managing stress and anxiety.

Support systems: family, friends, and mental health professionals

Support systems, including family, friends, and mental health professionals, are invaluable resources for individuals dealing with challenges such as Polycystic Ovary Syndrome (PCOS) or any other stressors in life. These support networks play a significant role in providing emotional assistance, guidance, and understanding. Here's how each type of support system can contribute to your well-being:

1. Family Support:
- Family members can offer unconditional love, understanding, and a sense of belonging.
- They can provide practical assistance, such as helping with daily tasks, accompanying you to appointments, or offering childcare.
- Communicate openly with your family about your needs, feelings, and challenges, so they can offer appropriate support.

2. Friendships:
- Friends can provide companionship, a listening ear, and a sense of normalcy during difficult times.
- They can offer different perspectives, advice, and empathy from their own experiences.

- Maintain open communication with friends and let them know how they can support you effectively.

3. Mental Health Professionals:
- Mental health professionals, such as therapists, counselors, and psychologists, specialize in providing support for emotional challenges.
- They can offer coping strategies, teach relaxation techniques, and help you work through difficult emotions.
- Seeking professional help can offer a safe space to discuss your concerns and receive expert guidance.

4. Benefits of Support Systems:
- Emotional Outlet: Support systems provide a safe space to express your feelings, fears, and concerns without judgment.
- Validation: Being heard and understood by loved ones and professionals can validate your emotions and experiences.
- Perspective: Family, friends, and mental health professionals can offer different

perspectives that help you see situations from various angles.
- Coping Strategies: Support systems can share coping strategies, offer advice, and suggest techniques to manage stress and anxiety.
- Reduction of Isolation: Connecting with others reduces feelings of isolation and loneliness, creating a sense of belonging.

5. Building and Nurturing Support Systems:
- Communicate: Openly express your needs and feelings to your support network. Let them know how they can help you.
- Seek Professional Help: Don't hesitate to consult a mental health professional if you need specialized assistance.
- Mutual Support: Offer support to your loved ones when they need it as well. Relationships are a two-way street.

Remember that reaching out for support is a sign of strength, not weakness. Everyone needs assistance at times, and building a strong support network can help you navigate challenges with resilience and improve your overall well-being.

Building resilience and maintaining a positive outlook

Building resilience and maintaining a positive outlook are essential skills that can help individuals navigate challenges, including those posed by conditions like Polycystic Ovary Syndrome (PCOS). Resilience enables you to bounce back from setbacks and manage stressors more effectively. Here's how to build resilience and cultivate a positive outlook:

1. Develop Self-Awareness:
- Understand your strengths, weaknesses, and triggers. This self-awareness can help you manage challenges more effectively.

2. Optimism and Positive Thinking:
- Focus on the positive aspects of situations and practice reframing negative thoughts into more constructive ones.

3. Mindfulness and Present Moment Awareness:

- Practice mindfulness to stay present and reduce anxiety about the past or future. It can help you navigate challenges with a clear mind.

4. Problem-Solving Skills:

- Develop problem-solving skills to approach challenges with a proactive mindset. Break problems into smaller, manageable steps.

5. Healthy Lifestyle:

- Prioritize a balanced diet, regular exercise, sufficient sleep, and stress management to build physical and emotional resilience.

6. Seek Social Support:

- Connect with family, friends, or support groups. Sharing experiences and feelings can provide emotional relief and a sense of belonging.

7. Adaptability:

- Embrace change as an opportunity for growth rather than a threat. Flexibility can help you navigate unexpected challenges.

8. Set Realistic Goals:
- Break down your goals into achievable steps. Celebrate progress, no matter how small.

9. Humor and Laughter:
- Engage in activities that make you laugh. Laughter can be a powerful tool for reducing stress.

10. Acceptance:
- Accept that setbacks and challenges are a normal part of life. Focus on what you can control and let go of what you can't.

11. Self-Care:
- Prioritize self-care activities that promote relaxation and well-being, such as meditation, hobbies, or spending time in nature.

12. Seek Professional Help:

- If challenges become overwhelming, seek support from mental health professionals who can offer guidance and coping strategies.

13. Gratitude Practice:
- Focus on what you're grateful for. Gratitude can shift your perspective and improve your overall outlook.

14. Learn from Adversity:
- View challenges as opportunities for learning and growth. Overcoming obstacles can make you more resilient.

15. Embrace Mistakes:
- See mistakes as learning experiences, not failures. They contribute to personal growth.

Building resilience and maintaining a positive outlook are ongoing practices. By cultivating these skills, you'll be better equipped to navigate the ups and downs of life, including managing the challenges associated with PCOS or any other condition. Remember that small steps can lead to significant improvements in your overall well-being.

Chapter 9: PCOS-Related Health Risks

Long-term health risks: cardiovascular issues, diabetes, and more

Individuals with Polycystic Ovary Syndrome (PCOS) may be at a higher risk for certain long-term health issues, including cardiovascular issues, type 2 diabetes, and other metabolic concerns. It's important to be aware of these risks and take proactive steps to manage your health. Here's an overview of these potential long-term health risks and how to address them:

1. Cardiovascular Issues:

- Women with PCOS have an increased risk of cardiovascular diseases, including heart disease and stroke.
- Risk factors such as insulin resistance, obesity, and high blood pressure contribute to this increased risk.
- Manage your weight through a balanced diet and regular exercise to reduce cardiovascular risk factors.
- Monitor blood pressure and cholesterol levels regularly, and consult your healthcare provider for appropriate interventions if needed.

2. Type 2 Diabetes:
- Insulin resistance, a common feature of PCOS, increases the risk of developing type 2 diabetes.
- Focus on maintaining a healthy weight, following a balanced diet, and staying physically active to improve insulin sensitivity.
- Regular blood sugar monitoring is essential to detect any abnormalities early.

3. Metabolic Syndrome:

- Metabolic syndrome is a cluster of conditions that include high blood pressure, high blood sugar, excess abdominal fat, and abnormal cholesterol levels.
- Addressing underlying factors such as insulin resistance and weight management can help prevent or manage metabolic syndrome.

4. Endometrial Cancer:
- Women with PCOS may be at a slightly higher risk of developing endometrial (uterine) cancer due to irregular menstrual cycles and hormonal imbalances.
- Regular gynecological check-ups and discussions with your healthcare provider can help monitor and manage this risk.

5. Sleep Apnea:
- PCOS is associated with a higher risk of obstructive sleep apnea, a condition that affects breathing during sleep.
- Maintaining a healthy weight, sleeping in a comfortable position, and seeking medical treatment if needed can help manage sleep apnea.

6. Psychological and Emotional Well-being:
- Long-term health risks also extend to psychological well-being. Individuals with PCOS may experience anxiety, depression, and reduced quality of life.
- Prioritize mental health through self-care, social support, and seeking professional help when needed.

7. Regular Check-ups:
- Schedule regular medical check-ups to monitor your health, especially if you have PCOS or are at increased risk for related conditions.

8. Holistic Approach:
- Taking a holistic approach to health, including balanced nutrition, regular exercise, stress management, and adequate sleep, can significantly reduce these long-term health risks.

It's important to remember that everyone's health journey is unique. Consult with your healthcare provider to assess your individual risk factors and develop a personalized plan for managing your long-term health. By being proactive and making healthy lifestyle choices, you can significantly reduce the impact of these potential health risks associated with PCOS.

Regular health check-ups and monitoring

Regular health check-ups and monitoring are crucial for individuals with Polycystic Ovary Syndrome (PCOS) to ensure early detection, prevention, and effective management of potential health issues. Consistent medical assessments and monitoring can help you stay on top of your health, identify any emerging problems, and take timely action. Here's why regular check-ups and monitoring are important and what you should consider:

1. Early Detection and Prevention:
- Regular check-ups allow healthcare providers to identify health concerns early, increasing the likelihood of successful treatment and prevention of complications.

- Monitoring can help catch any deviations from normal health trends and enable prompt intervention.

2. PCOS-Related Risks:
- Regular monitoring is especially important for managing conditions associated with PCOS, such as insulin resistance, diabetes, cardiovascular issues, and hormonal imbalances.

3. Individualized Care:
- Healthcare providers can tailor their advice and recommendations based on your health status and specific needs.
- Personalized care can optimize your PCOS management and address any unique concerns.

4. Health Status Tracking:
- Regular monitoring helps track progress and the effectiveness of lifestyle changes, medications, or interventions you might be undergoing.

5. Comprehensive Assessments:
- Health check-ups provide a comprehensive assessment of your overall well-being, including physical, mental, and emotional health.

6. Peace of Mind:
- Regular health check-ups can provide reassurance about your health status, reduce anxiety, and offer a sense of control.

7. Recommendations for Action:
- Healthcare providers can offer guidance on managing symptoms, adjusting treatment plans, and making lifestyle modifications based on your health data.

8. Frequency of Check-ups:
- The frequency of check-ups depends on factors such as your age, health status, and specific conditions. Typically, annual check-ups are recommended, but individuals with PCOS may benefit from more frequent visits.

9. Collaboration with Healthcare Providers:
- Establish a collaborative relationship with your healthcare providers, including an OB/GYN, endocrinologist, and any other specialists as needed.
- Share your PCOS history, concerns, and any changes you've noticed since your last visit.

10. Self-Monitoring:
- Keep track of your menstrual cycles, blood pressure, blood sugar levels (if applicable), and any symptoms you experience between check-ups.

Remember that regular check-ups are an essential component of proactive healthcare. By staying engaged with your healthcare providers and staying diligent about monitoring your health, you can effectively manage your PCOS and minimize the potential long-term health risks associated with the condition.

Strategies for minimizing risks through lifestyle changes

Lifestyle changes play a significant role in minimizing the risks associated with Polycystic Ovary Syndrome (PCOS) and promoting overall well-being. By adopting healthy habits, individuals with PCOS can manage symptoms, improve metabolic health, and reduce the risk of long-term health complications. Here are strategies for minimizing risks through lifestyle changes:

1. Balanced Nutrition:
- Consume a balanced diet rich in whole foods, lean proteins, vegetables, fruits, whole grains, and healthy fats.
- Limit refined carbohydrates, sugars, and processed foods that can contribute to insulin resistance.
- Monitor portion sizes to prevent overeating and maintain a healthy weight.

2. Regular Exercise:
- Engage in regular physical activity, including both aerobic exercises (such as walking, jogging, or swimming) and strength training.

- Aim for at least 150 minutes of moderate-intensity exercise per week, with a mix of cardio and strength exercises.

3. Weight Management:
- Maintain a healthy weight through a combination of a balanced diet and regular exercise.
- Weight loss, even a modest amount, can improve insulin sensitivity and reduce PCOS symptoms.

4. Stress Management:
- Practice stress reduction techniques such as meditation, deep breathing, yoga, or mindfulness.
- Reducing stress can help manage hormonal imbalances and improve overall well-being.

5. Sleep Hygiene:
- Prioritize quality sleep by establishing a regular sleep schedule and creating a comfortable sleep environment.
- Aim for 7-9 hours of uninterrupted sleep each night.

6. Regular Monitoring:
- Monitor key health indicators such as blood pressure, blood sugar levels (if applicable), cholesterol levels, and weight.
- Regular monitoring helps track your progress and identify any deviations from normal ranges.

7. Avoid Smoking and Limit Alcohol:
- Quit smoking, as smoking can worsen metabolic and cardiovascular risks.
- If you choose to drink alcohol, do so in moderation and within recommended guidelines.

8. Hydration:
- Drink plenty of water throughout the day to stay hydrated and support overall health.

9. Consistent Meal Timing:
- Eat regular meals and snacks at consistent intervals to stabilize blood sugar levels and manage insulin resistance.

10. Support System:

- Build a strong support system through friends, family, and support groups to provide encouragement and accountability.

11. Regular Medical Check-ups:
- Schedule regular medical check-ups with your healthcare providers to monitor your health, discuss progress, and adjust strategies if needed.

12. Professional Guidance:
- Consult healthcare professionals, including a registered dietitian, fitness expert, or mental health professional, for personalized guidance tailored to your needs.

Remember that making lifestyle changes is a gradual process, and consistency is key. Small, sustainable changes over time can have a significant positive impact on your overall health and well-being. Working with healthcare professionals and involving your support network can further enhance your efforts to minimize risks associated with PCOS.

Chapter 10: Research and Future Directions

Current scientific research on PCOS

1. Genetic Studies: Researchers were continuing to explore the genetic factors contributing to PCOS. Identifying specific genes and genetic variations associated with the condition could provide insights into its underlying mechanisms.

2. Hormonal and Metabolic Pathways: Studies were investigating the intricate interplay between hormonal imbalances, insulin resistance, and the development of PCOS. Understanding these pathways could lead to targeted treatments.

3. Gut Microbiome: Research was exploring the potential link between gut health and PCOS. Emerging evidence suggested that alterations in the gut microbiome might influence metabolic health and PCOS symptoms.

4. Inflammation and Immune System: Investigations were underway to determine the role of chronic inflammation and immune system dysfunction in PCOS. Inflammation might contribute to insulin resistance and other PCOS-related issues.

5. Lifestyle Interventions: Researchers were examining the effects of various lifestyle modifications, including diet, exercise, and stress management, on PCOS symptoms and overall health.

6. Cardiovascular Risks: Studies were looking into the increased risk of cardiovascular diseases among individuals with PCOS. This included assessing the impact of PCOS on lipid profiles, blood pressure, and other cardiovascular markers.

7. Fertility Treatments: Research focused on improving fertility treatments for women with PCOS, including advancements in assisted reproductive technologies and tailored approaches to ovulation induction.

8. Mental Health: Studies were investigating the psychological impact of PCOS, including the prevalence of anxiety, depression, and other mental health concerns among individuals with the condition.

For the most up-to-date and comprehensive information on current scientific research on PCOS, I recommend checking reputable medical journals, university research websites, and sources like the National Institutes of Health (NIH) or medical databases such as PubMed. Keep in mind that research is an ongoing process, and new discoveries are made regularly that can shape our understanding and management of PCOS.

Emerging treatments and interventions

There are several emerging treatments and interventions being explored for Polycystic Ovary Syndrome (PCOS). Keep in mind that medical research is an ongoing process, and developments have occurring since then.

Here are some areas that were being investigated:

1. Precision Medicine: Researchers were studying personalized treatment approaches based on an individual's genetic makeup, hormonal profile, and other factors. Tailoring interventions to each person's unique characteristics could lead to more effective treatments.

2. Anti-Inflammatory Therapies: Inflammation was being recognized as a potential contributor to PCOS symptoms. Studies were exploring the effects of anti-inflammatory medications and lifestyle changes in managing inflammation and its impact on PCOS.

3. Gut Microbiome Modulation: Some research suggested a connection between the gut microbiome and PCOS. Investigating ways to modulate the gut microbiome through diet, prebiotics, probiotics, and other interventions could have implications for PCOS management.

4. Insulin-Sensitizing Agents: While medications like metformin have been used to improve insulin sensitivity, new agents were being investigated to address insulin resistance more effectively and with fewer side effects.

5. Targeted Hormonal Therapies: Researchers were exploring novel hormonal treatments that could more specifically target the underlying hormonal imbalances in PCOS while minimizing unwanted side effects.

6. Nutritional Approaches: Studies were examining the effects of specific diets and nutritional supplements on PCOS symptoms. Low-glycemic diets, Mediterranean diets, and certain supplements were under investigation.

7. Exercise Interventions: Research was focusing on the type, duration, and intensity of exercise that could be most beneficial for managing PCOS-related issues, such as insulin resistance and weight management.

8. Behavioral Interventions: Behavioral therapies, including cognitive-behavioral therapy and mindfulness-based interventions, were being studied for their potential to address psychological symptoms and improve overall well-being.

9. Ovulation Induction Innovations: Advancements were being made in assisted reproductive technologies, including improved protocols for ovulation induction and in vitro fertilization (IVF) tailored to the needs of women with PCOS.

10. Telemedicine and Digital Health: With the growth of telemedicine and digital health platforms, researchers were exploring the feasibility and effectiveness of remote interventions for PCOS management, including virtual consultations, apps, and online support groups.

For the latest updates on emerging treatments and interventions for PCOS, I recommend checking reputable medical journals, academic research institutions, and organizations dedicated to PCOS research and advocacy. Consulting with a healthcare provider knowledgeable about the latest research developments can also provide valuable insights.

Advocacy and awareness initiatives

Advocacy and awareness initiatives for Polycystic Ovary Syndrome (PCOS) are crucial for increasing understanding, promoting research, and supporting individuals affected by the condition. These initiatives aim to raise awareness among the public, healthcare professionals, policymakers, and the media about the challenges faced by individuals with PCOS. Here are some ways advocacy and awareness efforts are conducted:

1. Education and Information Dissemination:
- Develop educational materials, websites, and resources to provide accurate information about PCOS, its symptoms, causes, and available treatments.

- Organize webinars, workshops, and conferences to educate healthcare providers, patients, and the general public.

2. Support Networks and Communities:
- Establish support groups, both in-person and online, where individuals with PCOS can share experiences, advice, and emotional support.
- Provide a platform for individuals to connect with others facing similar challenges.

3. Media and Social Media Campaigns:
- Use social media platforms, blogs, and podcasts to share stories, dispel myths, and raise awareness about PCOS.
- Launch campaigns during PCOS Awareness Month (September) to bring attention to the condition.

4. Advocacy for Research Funding:
- Advocate for increased funding for PCOS research to better understand its causes, improve treatments, and develop more effective interventions.

5. Collaboration with Healthcare Professionals:
- Collaborate with healthcare providers to enhance their understanding of PCOS, improving diagnosis and treatment options.

6. Government Engagement:
- Lobby policymakers to prioritize PCOS on public health agendas, advocating for research funding, improved diagnostic criteria, and support programs.

7. Awareness Events:
- Organize walks, runs, and other events to raise funds for research and increase community engagement.
- Collaborate with local organizations, schools, and institutions to host awareness events.

8. Research Initiatives:
- Support and promote research studies to better understand PCOS and its implications, such as its impact on mental health, fertility, and long-term health.

9. Partnerships:
- Collaborate with medical organizations, universities, healthcare providers, and other stakeholders to collectively raise awareness and support research efforts.

10. Empowerment and Advocacy Training:
- Provide resources and training for individuals with PCOS to become advocates and empower them to share their stories effectively.

By raising awareness and advocating for PCOS, these initiatives help reduce stigma, improve diagnosis and treatment, and provide individuals with the support and resources they need to manage the condition effectively. If you're interested in getting involved, consider joining or supporting established PCOS advocacy organizations or starting your own awareness campaigns in your community.

The road ahead: hope for women with PCOS

The road ahead holds much hope for women with Polycystic Ovary Syndrome (PCOS). Advances in research, increased awareness, and improved healthcare approaches are offering a brighter outlook for those affected by the condition. Here are some reasons for hope:

1. Improved Understanding: Ongoing research is deepening our understanding of PCOS, shedding light on its underlying causes, genetic factors, and complex interactions. This understanding is leading to more targeted treatments and interventions.

2. Personalized Treatment: With the rise of precision medicine, treatments are becoming more tailored to individual needs. This means more effective management of PCOS symptoms and a better quality of life for each person.

3. Lifestyle Management: The power of lifestyle changes in managing PCOS is gaining recognition. Women have the tools to

make positive changes in their diet, exercise, and stress management to improve their health and well-being.

4. Mental Health Focus: Awareness is growing about the psychological impact of PCOS. As mental health becomes an integral part of PCOS care, support and treatment for anxiety, depression, and stress are becoming more accessible.

5. Fertility Advancements: Assisted reproductive techniques are continually advancing, offering better chances of conception for women with PCOS who face fertility challenges.

6. Comprehensive Care: Healthcare providers are increasingly adopting a multidisciplinary approach to PCOS care, addressing not only the physical symptoms but also emotional well-being, mental health, and overall quality of life.

7. Advocacy and Support: PCOS advocacy organizations are working tirelessly to raise

awareness, reduce stigma, and provide resources and support for women with PCOS. Their efforts are helping create a more informed and empowered community.

8. Patient Empowerment: Women with PCOS are taking charge of their health by seeking information, advocating for themselves, and actively participating in their treatment plans. This empowerment is fostering positive changes in how PCOS is managed.

9. Future Research: Ongoing and future research may reveal even more about PCOS, leading to breakthroughs in treatment, prevention, and potentially even a better understanding of how to manage its long-term health risks.

10. Community and Connection: The sense of community among women with PCOS is growing stronger. Online forums, support groups, and social media platforms provide spaces for sharing experiences, seeking advice, and finding solidarity.

With each passing year, our collective understanding of PCOS is expanding, and new tools and resources are emerging to support those affected. The road ahead is one of hope, progress, and empowerment for women with PCOS as they navigate their health journeys with resilience and determination.

Epilogue: Empowered Living with PCOS

The journey of embracing one's body and health

Embracing one's body and health is a profound and transformative journey, especially for individuals dealing with conditions like Polycystic Ovary Syndrome (PCOS). This journey involves developing a positive relationship with your body, fostering self-acceptance, and prioritizing your well-being. Here are some steps you can take on this journey:

1. Self-Compassion:

- Practice self-compassion by treating yourself with the same kindness and understanding you would offer a friend. Be patient with your body and acknowledge that it's doing its best.

2. Mindful Awareness:
- Cultivate mindfulness by paying attention to your body's signals, sensations, and needs without judgment. Mindful practices can help you appreciate your body's strengths and listen to its cues.

3. Shift Your Perspective:
- Focus on what your body can do rather than how it looks. Celebrate your body's functionality, strength, and resilience.

4. Set Realistic Goals:
- Set achievable health and fitness goals that are not solely centered around appearance. Prioritize goals that enhance your overall well-being and self-esteem.

5. Challenge Negative Thoughts:

- When negative thoughts about your body arise, challenge them. Replace them with positive affirmations and gratitude for your body's abilities.

6. Nourishing Self-Care:
- Engage in self-care activities that make you feel good both physically and mentally. These can include relaxing baths, engaging in hobbies, or spending time in nature.

7. Surround Yourself Positively:
- Surround yourself with people who support and uplift you. Minimize exposure to negative influences that might hinder your journey.

8. Celebrate Progress:
- Acknowledge and celebrate small victories in your health journey. Every step forward is a success worth celebrating.

9. Seek Professional Guidance:
- If struggling with body image issues, consider speaking to a mental health

professional who specializes in body positivity and self-esteem.

10. Let Go of Perfectionism:
- Embrace imperfections as part of being human. Recognize that nobody's body is perfect, and that's okay.

11. Focus on Health, Not Weight:
- Shift your focus from weight to overall health. Prioritize nutritious foods, regular exercise, and stress management for your well-being.

12. Practice Gratitude:
- Cultivate gratitude for your body's abilities and resilience. This can help shift your mindset toward a more positive outlook.

**13. Embrace Imperfections:
- Accept that your body may change over time due to various factors, and that's part of life's journey.

Remember that embracing your body and health is an ongoing process, and it's okay to have both good and challenging days. By treating yourself with kindness, respecting your body, and prioritizing your overall well-being, you can embark on a transformative journey of self-acceptance and empowerment.

Success stories of women managing PCOS

There are countless inspiring success stories of women who have effectively managed Polycystic Ovary Syndrome (PCOS) and have taken charge of their health and well-being. These stories highlight the resilience, determination, and positive changes that individuals can achieve. Here are a few success stories to inspire you:

*1. Emma's Journey to a Balanced Lifestyle:**
Emma struggled with weight gain, insulin resistance, and irregular periods due to PCOS. She decided to take control of her health by adopting a balanced diet rich in whole foods, practicing regular exercise, and managing stress through yoga and meditation. Over time, Emma lost weight, improved her

insulin sensitivity, and her menstrual cycles became more regular. She now shares her journey on social media to inspire others to make positive changes.

**2. Sarah's Fertility Triumph:
Sarah faced challenges conceiving due to PCOS-related ovulatory dysfunction. With guidance from her healthcare provider, she started medication to induce ovulation and adopted a healthy lifestyle. After a few months, Sarah successfully conceived and gave birth to a healthy baby. Her story highlights the potential for successful pregnancies with the right interventions and lifestyle changes.

3. Jenny's Journey to Emotional Well-being:
Jenny struggled with mood swings, anxiety, and depression alongside her PCOS symptoms. She decided to prioritize her mental health by seeking therapy, practicing mindfulness, and engaging in hobbies she enjoyed. Over time, Jenny found her emotional well-being improving, and she developed effective coping strategies to

manage both her PCOS and her mental health.

4. Maria's Positive Body Image Transformation:
Maria faced body image issues and struggled with self-acceptance due to PCOS-related weight changes. Through counseling, self-compassion exercises, and surrounding herself with supportive friends, she underwent a transformation in her self-perception. Maria now embraces her body as it is and focuses on its strength and abilities rather than its appearance.

5. Lily's Journey to Hormonal Balance:
Lily's PCOS caused irregular periods, acne, and excessive hair growth. She worked closely with her healthcare provider to develop a tailored treatment plan. Lily incorporated dietary changes, regular exercise, and hormone-balancing medications. Over time, her symptoms improved significantly, and she gained a better understanding of her body's needs.

These success stories demonstrate that with determination, self-care, professional guidance, and the right strategies, women can make positive changes in their lives despite the challenges of PCOS. Each journey is unique, and what works for one person might differ for another. The key is to find a personalized approach that aligns with your goals and needs, leading you to improved health and overall well-being.

Final thoughts on resilience, self-care, and advocacy

Here are some final thoughts on resilience, self-care, and advocacy for individuals dealing with Polycystic Ovary Syndrome (PCOS):

Resilience:
- Resilience is the ability to adapt and thrive despite challenges. PCOS can present various obstacles, but cultivating resilience allows you to navigate them with strength and determination.

- Remember that setbacks are a normal part of any journey. It's how you respond and persevere that truly defines your resilience.
- Seek support from friends, family, and support groups. Connecting with others who understand your experiences can provide comfort and encouragement.

Self-Care:
- Self-care isn't selfish; it's essential for your well-being. Prioritize self-care activities that nourish your mind, body, and soul.
- Listen to your body's needs. Rest when you're tired, nourish yourself with healthy foods, and engage in activities that bring you joy.
- Practice self-compassion. Treat yourself with kindness and understanding, just as you would a friend facing challenges.

Advocacy:
- Advocacy is about raising awareness, making your voice heard, and driving positive change.
- Be an advocate for your own health. Educate yourself about PCOS, ask questions

during medical appointments, and actively participate in your treatment decisions.
- Consider becoming an advocate within the PCOS community. Share your story, engage in awareness campaigns, and support efforts to improve understanding and research.

Remember that your journey with PCOS is unique, and it's okay to ask for help when needed. Embrace the lessons, celebrate your successes, and keep moving forward with resilience, self-care, and advocacy as your guiding principles. Your strength and determination can inspire not only yourself but also others facing similar challenges.

APPENDICES

Glossary of medical terms related to PCOS

Sure, here's a glossary of some common medical terms related to Polycystic Ovary Syndrome (PCOS):

1. **Polycystic Ovary Syndrome (PCOS):** A hormonal disorder characterized by irregular menstrual cycles, excess androgen levels, and the presence of cysts on the ovaries.

2. **Androgens:** Male hormones, such as testosterone, that are present in both males and females but are typically at lower levels in females.

3. **Insulin Resistance:** A condition where the body's cells do not respond

effectively to insulin, leading to elevated blood sugar levels and potentially contributing to PCOS.

4. **Hirsutism:** Excessive hair growth in areas where it's typically seen in males, such as the face, chest, and back, due to elevated androgen levels.

5. **Amenorrhea:** The absence of menstrual periods for an extended period, often due to hormonal imbalances.

6. **Anovulation:** Lack of ovulation or failure to release a mature egg from the ovaries during the menstrual cycle.

7. **Oligomenorrhea:** Infrequent or irregular menstrual periods, often characterized by cycles longer than 35 days.

8. **Hyperandrogenism:** Excessive levels of androgens (male hormones) in the body, leading to symptoms like acne, hirsutism, and male-pattern hair loss.

9. **Menstrual Cycle:** The regular series of changes in the female reproductive system that prepares the body for pregnancy.

10. **Follicles:** Fluid-filled sacs within the ovaries that contain immature eggs. In PCOS, these follicles may not mature properly, leading to cyst formation.

11. **Metabolic Syndrome:** A cluster of conditions that include obesity, high blood pressure, insulin resistance, and abnormal lipid levels, increasing the risk of cardiovascular diseases.

12. **Endometrial Hyperplasia:** An overgrowth of the uterine lining due to hormonal imbalances, potentially increasing the risk of endometrial cancer.

13. **Gestational Diabetes:** Diabetes that develops during pregnancy due to insulin resistance.

14. **Luteinizing Hormone (LH):** A hormone that triggers ovulation and the release of the mature egg from the ovary.

15. **Follicle-Stimulating Hormone (FSH):** A hormone that stimulates the growth and development of follicles in the ovaries.

16. **Thyroid-Stimulating Hormone (TSH):** A hormone that regulates the thyroid gland's production of hormones, which influence metabolism and other bodily functions.

17. **Glucose Tolerance Test:** A test used to diagnose diabetes and insulin resistance by measuring blood sugar levels before and after consuming a glucose solution.

18. **Insulin Sensitizers:** Medications used to improve the body's response to insulin and manage insulin resistance.

19. **Ovulation Induction:** Medical intervention to stimulate ovulation in women who are not ovulating regularly.

20. **Assisted Reproductive Techniques (ART):** Medical procedures, including in vitro fertilization (IVF), used to help individuals or couples conceive when natural methods are not effective.

Resources for further information, support groups, and online communities

Certainly, here are some resources, support groups, and online communities where you can find further information and connect with others dealing with Polycystic Ovary Syndrome (PCOS):

Websites and Organizations:
1. **PCOS Challenge:** A nonprofit organization that offers education, support, and advocacy for individuals with PCOS. Website: [pcoschallenge.org](https://www.pcoschallenge.org/)

2. **PCOS Awareness Association:** A resource hub for PCOS information, awareness, and support. Website: [pcosaa.org](https://www.pcosaa.org/)

3. **The Center for Young Women's Health:** Provides reliable health

information for young women, including comprehensive information on PCOS. Website: youngwomenshealth.org

4. **Mayo Clinic PCOS Information:** Offers comprehensive information about PCOS, its symptoms, causes, and treatments. Website: [mayoclinic.org](https://www.mayoclinic.org/diseases-conditions/pcos/)

Online Communities and Support Groups:
1. **Soul Cysters:** An online community and support forum for women with PCOS to share experiences, ask questions, and find understanding. Website: [soulcysters.net](https://www.soulcysters.net/)

2. **My PCOS Team:** An online platform where individuals with PCOS can connect, share advice, and support each other. Website:

[mypcosteam.com](https://www.mypcosteam.com/)

3. **Reddit PCOS Community:** A subreddit where individuals with PCOS discuss their experiences, share information, and provide support. Subreddit: [/r/PCOS](https://www.reddit.com/r/PCOS/)

Social Media Groups:
1. **PCOS Support on Facebook:** A group that offers a safe space for women to discuss their experiences with PCOS and provide support. Group: [PCOS Support](https://www.facebook.com/groups/pcossupport/)

2. **Instagram PCOS Community:** Search for hashtags like #PCOSCommunity, #PCOSAwareness, and #PCOSJourney to find inspiring stories and supportive accounts.

Remember that while online communities can provide valuable support and information, it's important to verify the credibility of the information you come across.

Sample meal plans and exercise routines

Here are sample meal plans and exercise routines that can be customized to your preferences and needs. Remember to consult with a healthcare professional before making significant changes to your diet or exercise routine, especially if you have any underlying health conditions.

Sample Meal Plans:

Day 1:
- Breakfast: Greek yogurt with berries and a sprinkle of nuts/seeds.
- Lunch: Grilled chicken salad with mixed greens, veggies, avocado, and a light vinaigrette.

- Snack: Carrot and cucumber sticks with hummus.
- Dinner: Baked salmon with quinoa and steamed broccoli.

Day 2:
- Breakfast: Oatmeal with sliced banana and almond butter.
- Lunch: Quinoa and black bean bowl with salsa, avocado, and mixed greens.
- Snack: Handful of almonds.
- Dinner: Stir-fried tofu with a variety of colorful veggies and brown rice.

Day 3:
- Breakfast: Whole-grain toast with scrambled eggs and spinach.
- Lunch: Lentil soup with a side salad.
- Snack: Greek yogurt with a drizzle of honey.
- Dinner: Grilled lean steak with sweet potato and roasted Brussels sprouts.
Sample Exercise Routines:

Day 1: Cardio and Strength Training

- Warm-up: 5 minutes of brisk walking or light jogging.
- Cardio: 20-30 minutes of brisk walking, jogging, or cycling.
- Strength Training: Bodyweight exercises (push-ups, squats, lunges, planks) for 20 minutes.
- Cool Down: Stretching for 5-10 minutes.

Day 2: Yoga and Flexibility
- Warm-up: 5 minutes of gentle stretching.
- Yoga: 30-40 minutes of a yoga routine focusing on flexibility and relaxation.
- Cool Down: 5-10 minutes of deep stretching.

Day 3: High-Intensity Interval Training (HIIT)
- Warm-up: 5 minutes of light cardio (jumping jacks, jogging in place).
- HIIT: Alternate between 30 seconds of high-intensity exercises (e.g., burpees, squat jumps) and 30 seconds of rest. Repeat for 20-25 minutes.
- Cool Down: 5-10 minutes of stretching.

Remember to adjust the intensity and duration of exercises based on your fitness level and any medical considerations. Consistency is key, and it's important to find exercises you enjoy and can sustain over time. Additionally, listen to your body, stay hydrated, and don't forget the importance of rest and recovery. If you're new to exercise, consider working with a fitness professional to ensure proper form and safety.

Medication reference guide

Here's a reference guide to common medications used for managing Polycystic Ovary Syndrome (PCOS). Please note that this guide provides general information, and you should always consult a healthcare professional before starting or adjusting any medication. Medications may have different names and formulations based on your location and healthcare provider's recommendations.

1. Oral Contraceptives (Birth Control Pills):
- Purpose: Regulate menstrual cycles, reduce androgen levels, manage acne and hirsutism.
- Examples: Yaz, Yasmin, Ortho Tri-Cyclen, Diane-35.

2. Anti-Androgens:
- Purpose: Reduce the effects of excess androgens, such as hirsutism and acne.
- Examples: Spironolactone, Cyproterone acetate (in combination with birth control pills).

3. Insulin-Sensitizing Medications:
- Purpose: Improve insulin sensitivity, manage insulin resistance, regulate menstrual cycles, and support fertility.
- Examples: Metformin, Glucophage, Pioglitazone.

4. Fertility Medications:
- Purpose: Induce ovulation in women who are not ovulating regularly.
- Examples: Clomiphene citrate, Letrozole.

5. Anti-Diabetic Medications:
- Purpose: Manage insulin resistance and improve blood sugar levels.
- Examples: Metformin (also used for PCOS-related insulin resistance), Acarbose.

6. Hormone Replacement Therapy (HRT):
- Purpose: Provide hormone replacement in postmenopausal women with PCOS to manage symptoms.
- Examples: Estrogen-progestin combinations.

7. Weight Management Medications:
- Purpose: Assist with weight loss and management, which can improve insulin sensitivity.
- Examples: Orlistat.

8. Hair Growth Inhibitors:
- Purpose: Slow down hair growth in hirsutism.

- Examples: Eflornithine cream.

Remember, PCOS treatment is highly individualized. Your healthcare provider will consider your specific symptoms, medical history, and goals when recommending medications. Always discuss potential side effects, benefits, and risks with your healthcare professional before starting any medication.